THE MUSICAL PAINTBOX

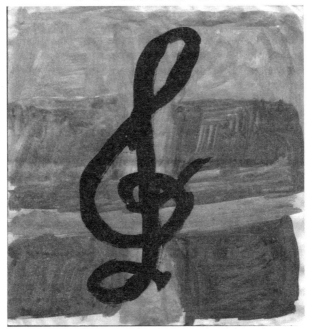

by Fiona Whelpton

One million people commit suicide every year.
The World Health Organization

1

Published by:
Chipmunka publishing
PO Box 6872
Brentwood
Essex
CM13 1ZT
United Kingdom

http://www.chipmunkapublishing.com

Copyright © 2006 Fiona Whelpton

ISBN 13:   978-1-905610-93-8

For Jason Pegler,
With much love, respect and gratitude

Also for Dolly Sen, and Sarah Tonin. All my love to Ollie
Frame, Creative Routes resident chef and admin worker,
thank you so much for all the gentle tender loving care, and
all my other mad brothers and sisters in Creative Routes
who inspire me with their creative subservience. It takes
special people to change the world. Here's to making the
mad voice heard.

Also thanks to Sue who has survived all the problems with
me through the years, I hope we will be there for each other
for many years to come.

Finally for Neil Arksey, you told me once that one could
grow through loss. This novel is (hopefully) testimony to
that. Thanks Neil for the inspiration.

Not forgetting the four-legged friends. In memory of Cup a
Soup, Pot Noodle, Creative Routes Agony Auntie, Lady
Gem Barker, Bluebell and Sascha, who keep their insane
pets sane.

Foreword:

The Musical Paintbox is a story which opens up like a
Pandora's Box of painful melodic writings. It is wonderful
prose that plays a poignant song in your head and paints a
touching sadness onto your heart. Each word, each note
has its own colour, its own emotion, and Fiona conducts it
beautifully in her writing. Listen, look and touch and this
book will both enchant and pain you in symphonic
tenderness. An exceptional read.

Dolly Sen

PROLOGUE

Pavane For A Dead Princess

Mrs Powell couldn't get away from the presence of the painting on the wall in her living room; it seemed to have a presence, which followed her about everywhere she went. She could feel eyes following her everywhere, with a piercing stare…

The picture evoked memories that she would have preferred not to remember. Evocative images, different angles, different aspects of her dead daughter's personality which would haunt her forever, constantly reminding her of her daughter's voice, the voice which had no voice, but had many voices.

Now it had gone beyond the voice, pushing the boundaries, so that the voices which had been stilled seemed to come back with a scream making their piercing presence felt in the picture of her daughter.

'I could have done so much more' Claire's mother agonised. 'But what more could I, or should I have done? Did I push Claire too far; push her over the edge – why didn't she feel listened to, when I always told her to come to us? I thought she wanted the piano more than anything else'

Mrs Powell knew she had not known her daughter. None of them had. None of them knew anything about her secret. They were family. It was their business to know, and they had failed miserably in their job as parents. They had completely failed. Claire, she must have felt so alone.

The tormenting thoughts kept returning. Mrs Powell removed the picture on the wall, hoping to get some peace. She put the picture in the attic. But it still haunted her. The guilt she felt was worse than the sense of inadequacy that she had felt since her daughter's death. She would never be free of it. She thought that somehow getting rid of the picture would help her find some peace of mind. But it didn't, it couldn't. The painting belonged on the wall. It was a god-given right. Something urged her to get the painting from the attic and put it back up. There was no escape, no place to go to, no place to run. The only place she had left was inside herself.

THE STUDENTS' HALL OF RESIDENCE
A Gruesome Discovery

The mystery begins to unfold…

It was the last week of the Christmas term. Everyone was too busy socialising, going out binge drinking, and to parties, to notice if any of their friends were missing. There was only one person who noticed…David, the artist. He was so similar to Claire. He'd feel lonely in a crowded room and out of place wherever he was unless there was a special person there too. When the other person was missing, he'd feel as if his whole world was empty, all of the time they were apart.

David had another unique gift, a sixth sense. He could tell when something was amiss through his intuition. He'd not seen Claire for a whole week, not since the end of term exams. He'd tried to include her in the various rounds of student parties, but there was no way of finding out where she'd gone…Or how to get hold of her. So he set himself a mission. But his journey led him to a terrible discovery.

The student caretaker found a body in one of the student's rooms. It was completely unidentifiable – so mutilated that they were unable to tell whether it was a young or old person. But David knew the answer, underneath, all the time; the truth was too painful for him to face up to. He didn't want to admit that the body was Claire's. How could it be, when she'd been so vibrant, and full of life? Now that life was over. There was a dark sense of death filling the air, and yet he could still sense Claire's very presence, even though he knew she'd left him forever. He didn't know how he was going to carry on without her…

PART 1
Frederick Chopin
The Raindrop Prelude

All Claire had ever wanted to do since she was a little girl was play the piano. That was her passion, her dream. She couldn't ever remember a time when she had ever wanted anything else as much, or more. In the end it became an obsession, which festered, and took hold of her. It became destructive. Destructive in such a way that she became embittered, as it eventually totally and utterly destroyed her. In the end, she would never play a single note ever again.

All those hours and hours and hours of endless practising – wasted. For what? What had happened was a complete mystery, even to people who considered that they had known her well – like David, the artist, who could see through Claire, the pianist, transparently. Suddenly, it seemed as if no one really knew her at all. Her closest friend, the artist, couldn't believe that he didn't remotely know her, and so he set out on a journey. A journey intended to piece together some of the missing parts of the unfinished jigsaw puzzle, whose pieces would all fit together in their correct position, in the end.

In order to be able to play to perfection and immerse herself in the magical world of sound, the musician needed solitude. Her fingers were able to run up and down the keyboard with ease, glorious harmonic progressions, the rippling arpeggios of Beethoven, the strong, firm, mighty passionate chords which require a woman to posses the strength of any man. But Claire was very much a person in her own right. She was not like the violinist, who needed other violinists in order to enlarge their sound, and needed to enlarge their sounds in order to embrace all the other stringed instruments of the orchestra. The chords of the piano were complete and perfect in their own right. From the major and minor chords of Beethoven to the whole tone scales of Debussy – the piano was very much its own

11

person. An empty room is easily filled with its grand presence without needing anyone, or anything else to embrace it.

The pianist needed to be alone, to be separate from other people, to be different, in order to perfect her art. But was it right to be alone in a room, for hours on end, solitary? Would it be possible for the pianist to be strong enough to be able to survive the isolation? On the outside she was strong enough but what was happening to her inner life? To her inner – being, which was somehow allowed to escape through the different colours and phrases of the sounds; the rising and falling of each melodic line as it merged into the phrases of each choral progression?

And what of the pianist, what made her tick and survive? There was something driving her, apart from the music. It wasn't just the power of the music by itself, it was an outside force. Most people need other people to survive. No one could survive with just the music for company. What made Claire survive if she was to at all?

The portrait was painted with every stroke of the brush, producing a different colour. The shape, form, and style all merged together to produce.

The Portrait of The Pianist

The Poppy Field

As her mother picked up the letters she saw that one of them was addressed to Claire, her daughter, who was expecting her 'A level' exam results. Her mother had her qualms about her daughter's grades. She knew that all Claire ever did with her life was work outrageously hard. Her daughter was a perfectionist. She had always had to prove to herself that she would achieve higher academic grades than any other student in her year. But she was different to the other students. She had an unusual, exceptional talent, which had emerged when Claire, who

12

was two years old at the time, had woken up the rest of the house by coming downstairs early in the morning to pick out tunes on the piano, before anyone else had even thought about waking up.

'The piano had always been Claire's passion,' thought Mrs Powell. But now passion wasn't exactly the right word to use to describe her daughter's obsession with music. Music consumed Claire's thoughts. Music came from every room in the house – Bach, Beethoven, Mozart, and then there were Claire's endless hours and hours and hours of practising. Mrs Powell was trying to help her daughter to hurry up, because she had at least an hour's piano practise to do before setting off to school, after breakfast.

The house would soon be filled with the sounds of scales and arpeggios running up and down the piano, each one needing to be memorised. Claire always started off a day's practising, at least an hour, with her technical exercises. Her scales were truly fluid, and her arpeggios flowed gracefully up and down the piano keyboard. But Mrs Powell knew that her daughter never believed that any of her playing was ever good enough – even though she worked herself like a Trojan.

Sometimes Claire's mother wondered whether her daughter was normal. It could hardly be considered normal behaviour for a teenager to cut herself off from all her school friends, and to have absolutely no social life at all – just because none of the others of her age had anything in common with her. Well, hopefully, Claire would be off to London to study music, and Mrs Powell was ever hopeful that her daughter's social life would improve as Claire had already found a place to live in a hostel for music students in Camberwell, South London, next to the Oval tube station, near Camberwell Green. It was for music students from all over London but there were plenty of pianos, so at least she wouldn't have the extra burden of struggling to find somewhere to practise. Claire had been studying for her final 'A level' exams and had had all the extra pressure of trying to mix her high powered practising with her revision.

Suddenly, alongside a normal teenager's existence Claire was finding her self-confidence had taken a massive tumble, and had reached the ultimate stages of an all time zero. She was agonising over prospective boyfriends (all of them who might show an interest in her, or torturing herself wondering if any of them would feel the same way about her as she did about them) She hated herself. Nothing about her life was right: her hair colour, eye colour and figure were all wrong. She always thought that she looked much too fat, and was on a permanent diet, but whatever the scales told her, she would never be satisfied.

Claire knew that she desperately needed to find something that would make her feel good about herself. But at this stage in her life, it seemed as if it was going to be impossible. The only positive thing she had in her life was her piano – at least she knew she was good at that. Even so, for all her perfectionism, lay a deep-rooted resentment and fear; a fear that no-one accepted her for who she was, people accepted and admired her for being gifted at her music but she could never be sure that anyone truly really liked her just the way she was, without having anything to prove.

'Because that's what the problem is all about, actually.' Claire mused to herself. 'I always need to prove myself to my parents, to my sister, and schoolmates. I always have to live up to their impossible expectations of me, that I am supposed to be exceptionally gifted. None of them have a clue that I am so utterly miserable.' She was right. No one had the slightest idea of the emotional turmoil that Claire went through every single day of her life.

Inside herself, she knew she was searching for something to relieve the burden. She thought that her music would help her to find creative fulfilment. But it was never enough. She looked for the fulfilment in her interaction with her peers, but amongst her acquaintances and friends there wasn't one single person whom she could relate her true feelings to. She needed to find one other person, a very special person – one of those people who knew exactly what she thought, someone she didn't need to talk to for hours on end without actually saying anything. Endless chatter – which actually meant nothing at all. Just words, empty words, bouncing backwards and forwards from the tongue, lashing out and bouncing around as if they were tennis balls. It just left the feeling that they were stone dead.

Leaving home and experiencing freedom for the first time had to be an important landmark in any normal eighteen year olds life. Mrs Powell however had high hopes that her daughter would find herself able to become like any other "normal" adolescent away from home. She would be forced to fend for herself. She often felt that she had failed her daughter as a mother. Even though Claire was extremely gifted – it still meant that she was something of an oddity, even thought of as a freak, by those who were in her peer group. It would have been so much easier had her daughter been exactly the same as any normal teenager – worrying about hairstyles, fashion, the latest images, and music. But Claire could hardly be called "normal." She just wasn't. In fact, there was nothing normal about her. She was distinctly abnormal, although these days, what the hell was normal, anyway?

The only thing in Claire's favour was her extremely strong sense of individuality, or so it appeared to those closest to her. But even those who thought they knew her intimately couldn't have had any indication that things were so badly wrong on the inside. How could they possibly, given that it was all one big game she was playing, trying to disguise her real self from the outside world?

The piano was her safety net. Without it, Claire had nothing extraordinary about her personality. Going away from home would be the only chance she'd get to prove to the world that she was her own person – someone who did not have to hide behind her music to win approval from others. Because she could be loved just for being who she was, without pretending to be something or somebody she wasn't, or couldn't ever hope to be. Claire needed a special friend to be with, to help her to discover those things, and that's how she came to know all there was to know about the artist, who was the only solitary person other than herself, who could possibly understand who she was, and what she was like. Claire had another secret, which no one else in the world could possibly know.

The Individual

Claire had stood out from the crowd ever since she had been in primary school. She hadn't joined in with the other children. Claire knew this was because she was shy, but the other children used to think of her as odd, eccentric, and they didn't want her in their group. She was always an observer – she never felt included.

The other girls in her class excelled in sport. Claire hated it passionately, but she was able to remain in control in a way that the others couldn't. She used her free periods to go to the school music block with special permission from the head teacher to use these lessons to do her practise. But her schoolmates always made fun of her being different. They hated her for it. They bullied her every single day. But she still needed her own private space. She was a born loner.

For some, individuality can prove to be a strength; individuality becomes a secret strength. No one could have guessed what was going on inside. The fact of the matter was that Claire didn't really know who she was at all. On reflection, as she looked back on her schooldays, the only memory she could recall was the taunting remarks and jeering faces of the playground. It was this that started to make her lose her self confidence, and she never really managed to regain her sense of self.

The answer to these problems was to lock herself away with her piano, her one comfort. But underneath was a deep dissatisfaction. One day Claire realised that she needed to find solace and become normal. The only way she could do this would be to break away from the expectations placed on her by her family to be somebody that she could never be.

Leaving home would give her the freedom that she had lacked. She could do what she wanted, whenever she liked, and more importantly, could be who she was without having to ask permission from her mother. Claire's mother thought she knew her daughter. The artist was the only person who managed to get a glimpse of the real person – the true self, or the motivation behind her true self.

Red poppies blazing in the golden sunshine in the case of the artist... The music and the schools in the case of the pianist... Bullying had endangered her life more than she really knew. The mysterious personality was never disclosed. But the artist set out to unlock the possibilities, and made it his quest to find out about the pianist. He was on a mission. But the results of the mission were completely surprising, and even Claire never realised there was a secret life, and the person she thought she was didn't really exist at all. But that was just part of the image...

David – The Artist

David was an art teacher at London University. He had been a professional artist before becoming involved in teaching art in order to support himself after his divorce had come through. He was a painter of rare talent. He'd been working hard, to be in a position to hold several exhibitions, but although his paintings were selling well, they weren't selling well enough to be able to make ends meet.

It seemed to be the answer to the loneliness that he had been experiencing after he had moved out of the family home, while his relationship with his wife was disintegrating. He had hardly realised how the relationship had suddenly

17

seemed to go downhill without him being conscious of the contributory factors. Everything had been like a whirlwind. One day his marriage was just the same as usual, the next day it seemed to have disintegrated so much that they didn't know what to do with each other. They were unable to communicate rationally, all because of a secret that had been going on for a good number of years, and had suddenly come right out into the open.

David had decided to spend much of his time travelling. It was during this time that he realized that what he really wanted to do was paint, watercolours and pastels. He was, however, exceptionally gifted at sketching portraits of his friends, and he had an exceptional gift of being able to see right through a person's individual character, and to be able to develop the person's real inner self. Whenever David would sketch a friend, he would spend a considerable amount of time with that person getting to know them properly. He would observe them, watch and listen to every mood swing, and would then choose the contrasting shades of dark and light – different colours to match the different moods.

David's idol was the French impressionist painter, Claude Monet, and his favourite painting was "The Poppy Field." Every time he looked at that painting, he felt as if he were in the middle of summer. He could almost feel the heat of the sunrays beating down on the green and yellow fields, ablaze with the magnificent scarlet-red poppies dancing in the breeze. Amsterdam was his favourite city, next to Paris. He loved its canals, waterways, and all the barges. The very pace of life slowed down by the waterside, which would automatically make his feel more rested. Amsterdam was also a safe haven for David's drug taking habit. He was able to indulge in it in a way that was more open than it was at home. In Amsterdam it was legal to smoke pot. In England it was a criminal offence to be found in possession of any kind of drug. So David was forced to keep his habit a secret. He had become an expert at lying to everybody. Firstly to his parents all the time he was growing up, since he'd been doing drugs whilst at school. They didn't have any idea about that part of his life. When he met Claire at university, he introduced them into her life too, and taught her how to keep their secrets. Until the day, that is, that Pandora's Box was opened. There were so many secrets let out of the box, each secret interwoven with another one, trying to conceal the ultimate secret of the secrecy to oneself. The discovery of each secret led to the ultimate self sacrifice.

It was David who made that fateful discovery. He and Claire had spent the previous evening together. She'd seemed to be her usual self, perfectly content and happy; David was now kicking himself for having got it so wrong. Then Claire started missing all her lectures, no one could make contact with her, so they turned to David, who they thought knew her better than anyone else. It was David who made the shocking discovery, which turned the student world upside down, forcing many of Claire's friends to grow up that year.

David wasn't so very different to Claire, which probably explained why she was able to open herself up to him. She opened herself up to him when he decided to paint a portrait of the most beautiful girl that he had ever seen in his life. Painting her became an opportunity for him to see the real person. She was completely exposed to him as he was painting her, so it wasn't surprising that she became transparent – that he began to gain a unique understanding of her – he could see beyond the person who kept herself separate from the rest of the world. He could tell perfectly well, so it was his right that he did become part of the jigsaw, that it was up to him to find that missing piece and put it right. It was Claire who discovered David's dark secret. It was Claire who discovered many of the artist's secrets. But she just accepted it, she wanted to help him, but in her desire to help she became swamped, got dragged into a situation that was way out of her depths.

The Sketch Of The Artist

It's time to meet David. The artist. We have just met him, but not properly, and that will be necessary, because it is always better to understand a person before condemning them for their inappropriate actions and behaviour without giving them a proper chance to reveal the real reason behind their behaviour. We are the ones who are the problem, in fact, when we decide to close doors against an individual who might be a bit different to the norm, because we have already made up our minds to turn our minds and hearts against them before we have even given them a proper chance. Letting them tell their story is a big part of that chance. Writing it for them gives them a chance to be able to be their true self, and to have their say. They sometimes need help to be able to tell the truth, because they have buried it too deeply into their subconscious to be able to deal with it properly. It is much more frightening to start to be honest with oneself. It takes real guts. Lots of it.

Loving another person makes this possible. If the other person is responsive to you, then you begin to feel safe enough to be your real person, without the need to pretend to be somebody else that you really aren't. That's when the cycle of stopping to feel out of sorts with oneself and the outside world can begin to be broken for good, and that one can begin a long healing process with the knowledge of the strength and warmth generating from another caring individual.

Real love can help hurting people blossom. Feeling accepted for who they are, without having to become like a performing monkey to win approval from society, or even other people in their family, who are often the main culprits, because they reduce the person into somebody who has insurmountable problems in their eyes – making them the black-sheep of their family, someone to be ashamed of.

A truly creative person not only has the ability to be able to use their art form to express their emotions but can also use it to bring healing into their broken lives rather than compounding the problem by burying deep-rooted anger into their sub-conscious and so not really confronting the real issues. A warm and close relationship with another understanding individual is often the one thing that the other person is lacking, so when chemistry happens between two artistically minded people it isn't surprising that it sparks off fireworks. Especially, when one of the individual's is going through the emotional up heave involved in the journey from childhood to adolescence, and then to adulthood. Sometimes the individual can appear to be more mature than they actually are. But the end result is catastrophic, because their emotions are not developed enough to be able to handle what's going on. The individual then becomes a wide-open target for experiencing mental health problems as a teenager. It is hardly surprising that most people start to experience mental health problems during their adolescence, given the communication difficulties experienced by most teenagers and their parents, even more so when the family is dysfunctional and unable to communicate without shouting. Artistic pursuits, music or visual arts seem to be the only way forward, and are the only answer.

Clouds Of Life, Nuages – Maurice Ravel

Melanie, David's wife, found that she was feeling as if she couldn't take any more. Communication between her and David were now fast becoming non-existent. It had got to the stage of a quick "hello" and "goodbye", when one or the other of them were going out of the front door in the mornings and with David not returning until she was already asleep in bed at night. These days, they couldn't really be called a family in a normal sense of the word. It was more a case of 'were you the person sitting behind the cornflakes packet this morning?' Melanie didn't even feel like a mother to her 14 year old daughter, Rosie, any longer, either. She was more like a carer than a mother. Rosie needed so much attention and looking after, Melanie felt that she was unable even to look after herself.

Rosie was the strange one – weird, peculiar, different, these were words that fitted her description perfectly. What made her weird was the fact that she would spend a great deal of time wandering off alone, talking to herself in long monologues, and then come back into the house saying that her voices had been telling her to do certain things. They were telling her that she was hopeless, giving her ideas about how to harm herself. She would not, or could not be comforted or reassured by anyone else. She was unable to connect with others. The only thing Melanie had felt able to do for her daughter was to make sure that she got her to the nearest accident and emergency department available. But the family was now becoming such frequent visitors there, that the staff saw them as nuisances, and refused to take them seriously any longer.

As she could no longer talk to her husband rationally about anything, Melanie was struggling with her own issues of anxiety, which would result in the occasional slanging matches with her daughter. So it was one particular day that Melanie had decided that it was high time that David pulled his head out of the sand, and listened to her, his wife, properly, for once. She decided to phone him on his mobile when he was still at work, but to no avail, of course. All she kept getting was the answer phone. She knew that she would have to make sure that she stayed awake long enough to ensure that they talked when he arrived back home from work that evening. But what was going to be the best way to get more than the occasional grunt from him, which was all he seemed to be capable of these days?

As Melanie mused over these thoughts while she was doing her ironing, there was a sudden tap on her front door. Putting her iron safely onto the stand, she went to answer the door, and found herself facing a policeman. Melanie knew in that split second, that something had happened to Rosie.
"What's happened?" Melanie asked.

"We want you to come to the hospital," replied the policeman. "It's your daughter, Rosie, isn't it? She's cut her wrists – somebody found her with blood pouring from them- sitting on the pavement in town. She refused to let them help her, so they called us, and I am afraid that we have had to section her, as she has a history of a personality disorder, and of hurting herself. She has quite a history of being uncooperative, doesn't she?" Melanie burst into tears "I had the feeling there was something wrong this morning" she said, "Just wait a minute, can you, while I get my coat."

She put it on as quickly as she could and followed the policeman, who escorted her into the waiting panda car. As she looked backwards at the house, she could see the neighbour's net curtains twitching. "The neighbours must be having a field-day," thought Melanie. "This will give them something interesting to gossip about. It would certainly liven up the conversation at the deathly boring Women's Institute tea party next week. But what's Rosie done to herself this time?"

The police arrived at the hospital, where they took Melanie to ask the waiting receptionist where she could find her daughter. The receptionist looked at her as if she were completely mad. "You were here last weekend," she said. "There isn't anything more we can do for your daughter. She is refusing help of any sort. I don't think that you should let her come home with you, either. She is obviously trying her best to manipulate you by hurting herself for no good reason. If she continues to refuse help there is nothing that anybody here can do for her. She is an attention-seeking time-waster who needs to be made to face up to life instead of running away from it all the time. You and your family don't help anything by pandering to all this attention seeking either, having her back home every time. She should be out on the streets."

"She's my daughter," said Melanie, coldly. "What am I supposed to do for her?"

"What's best for her is to be made to be independent," said the receptionist.

"Excuse me – but as her mother, don't I know what's best?" Melanie could feel herself becoming angrier and angrier. "You don't know her like I do."

"Of course, but anyone who tries to harm themselves without really intending to do too much serious damage, is doing it to manipulate somebody." replied the receptionist.

"You don't know what you are talking about." said Melanie not knowing how she had managed to stay as calm as she was "Did you know Rosie hears voices?"

"What do you mean?" asked the receptionist.

"Rosie hears voices, telling her unpleasant things all the time. She has schizophrenia. I think they tell her to hurt herself."

"I have never heard anything so ridiculous," said the receptionist. "All she's done this time is cut her wrists, and all we can do to help is to strap them up in bandages, take her to see the psychiatrist, which she always refuses to do – and send her home until the next time."

"I want to see my daughter," said Melanie firmly, "NOW"

"We've put her onto the psychiatric ward," said the receptionist "Follow the directions."

Every time Melanie had been to visit the acute psychiatric ward she had found it more and more traumatic. Everyone was like zombies in there; they didn't look like real people, even. You couldn't tell who they were. She couldn't even recognise Rosie. She had always had David with her, and felt supported by his strength, this time, however, she was alone, and she felt weak, vulnerable, and completely powerless to help her daughter to feel any better at all. Once she'd found the nurse in charge of the ward, the nurse had to locate Rosie. But she was only a student nurse, and didn't really even seem to know too much about where Rosie was.

"I thought that you were supposed to be making sure she was kept an eye on all the time" said a distraught Melanie. "What am I going to do?" Melanie appealed to the police officer standing at her side, looking as helpless as she felt. Melanie couldn't understand why the police seemed to be so inefficient "She has probably wandered off, like she does when this sort of thing happens. We must find her otherwise she'll end up being even more of a danger to herself than she already is."

"I'll go to look" offered the policeman "it's the least we can do for her seeing that we brought her all the way over here. Don't worry; she can't be very far away." He said, trying his best to reassure her.

"You don't know my daughter. If she chooses not to be found, she won't be found until she wants to be," replied Melanie.

"I think the best idea is for you to go back home and we'll call you as soon as we have found her..." ventured the policeman.

"Don't you think that it might be better if I'm here when you find her?" Melanie asked him, "after all, she's hardly likely to want to co-operate, she might even run off as soon as she sees the uniform."

"You have a point," he said. "Listen, then in that case why don't you have a cup of tea in the canteen, and they can come up to fetch you once we sort this out,"

"I can try to get hold of my husband, meanwhile" said Melanie. "Rosie is bound to be asking for him. She always prefers him than anybody else when this happens. He knows how to sort her out. At least one of us does." Melanie however had no idea that it was her husband that Rosie was running away from.

TWO MONTHS LATER

This last episode meant that Rosie had spent the longest period of time she'd ever done in the hospital. Melanie was never sure how useful it actually was to keep Rosie on an acute ward. She always seemed to cause disruption, with her attitude problem, and continually refused to accept that there was anything wrong with her. But this time, they seemed to have got it right. She'd finally managed to click with the member of staff they had chosen to be her key worker. Her name was Penny. Melanie liked her immediately. She was a grey-haired lady in her fifties, but was much more warm and caring than many of the psychiatric staff that Melanie had come into contact with on previous visits. There was something really caring about her placid nature and quiet manner, and Melanie had every faith that Rosie would respond to her immediately. She was perfect. Everybody's ideal nurse. Melanie had started worrying when she thought of some of the psychiatric staff they had had. She had always thought the staff used brute force when it came to dealing with their patients. She'd seen it time and again when they had arrived on a ward, the way they used more than one nurse to quieten what Melanie saw as a frightened person. The patient had every reason to be frightened too. Because the staff would make them feel completely intimidated. Why did they need to have more than one nurse helping a patient in acute distress? They were treated like criminals, just because they were in distress. It doesn't necessarily follow that they would be violent patients, but from the way they were treated by the staff, this was so often how the staff saw new admissions.

Melanie knew that she would be scared if she ever ended up having to be admitted onto a ward herself. The other patients were all so odd, that was enough to frighten anyone. Then there was the question of taking medication. No-one quite understood why some patients refused to take drugs; the side-effects were always there, and it seemed unfair to Melanie that patients weren't asked what they wanted, let alone listened to. She didn't feel good about not knowing where her daughter might be. So she took herself off to the hospital canteen. She felt very worried because she was convinced that Rosie was being plagued by the voices. This was usually the reason behind her getting lost, or wandering off on her own. Rosie would loose all sense of reality and time. To anyone on the outside, it seemed that she was talking to herself. But even though it seemed as if she was just talking to herself, she was actually participating in a very lively dialogue with these voices, which seemed set to be her tormentors, and made her life complete hell.

If Rosie had been able to keep a mobile with her, there might have at least have been some chance that Melanie could have made some contact with her, but she thought the voices were talking back to her through the phone, and refused to have one. All Melanie was able to do was to wait until the police called her down to the ward, as they had promised, but she didn't hold out too much hope.

ISOLATION

"Get AWAY from here...You have to get away, get away from here, get away from HERE. It's not safe, it's not safe, not safe, not safe..."The voices faded into the distance. Rosie felt relieved when she realised that they had eventually gone, but she had to get away from the police, and ambulance man – being in hospital made it worse, especially since the voices kept reminding her that it wasn't safe for her to be on the ward. But as soon as she had realised the voice had stopped, a new one, even harsher, louder, stared ringing in her ears. "They all want to hurt you, hurt you, hurt you, hurt you. David is going to get you, get you, get you, get YOU, get you, so GET OUT." "SHUT UP!!!!" Rosie screamed to the voices, at the top of her voice. But they didn't seem to want to hear her. They stayed with her, her tormentors. She had nowhere to run. No place of safety where she could get away to. The voices never faded into the distance. They were never background noises, just harsh permanent and tormenting voices. They drove Rosie to running away, going missing, because she was trying to run from the voices. But it turned into an endless game of 'Follow the leader'.

The every day noises of things going on around her couldn't even drown them out. Being in hospital made it worse. Then her psychiatrist came up with an answer to Rosie's dilemma. Rosie spent weeks hoping against hope that this would be the answer. But it was only the cause of a lot more problems. Rosie sincerely believed that the health service had let her down badly.

She felt she could never trust a psychiatrist ever again. These feelings of being unable to trust anything or anyone were enhanced by what the voices were trying to tell her through her delusions. Her psychiatrist had drawn the conclusion after many months of observation that she was an unsuitable case for psychotherapy but there might be a faint glimmer of hope for her if she would agree to have E.C.T. – Electric Convulsive Shock Therapy. This was supposed to get rid of the voices. But there were side effects attached to it. The psychiatrist didn't feel the patients were capable of making the right choices about having the treatment if they had all the facts.

Rosie would never have signed the consent forms had she been given the opportunity to investigate the full information about this treatment. Everyone has the right to find things out for themselves – don't they? Apparently not when you have a mental illness. The medical staff seem to think they have a god-given right to take your voices away from you. But there is never enough room for your own voice to be heard, loud and clear in the first place.

DEMORALISED is the one word that describes Rosie's place in society perfectly. DEMONISED is the way to describe the very same people who are supposed to be caring and treating psychiatric patients.

Rosie thought that there might be one sympathetic member of staff. This time Rosie was lucky in finding Penny, her key worker who liked her straight away, and the feeling was mutual. Rosie began to build the bridges of being able to trust somebody again. Penny's instincts would eventually tell her where Rosie could be found when she went missing. Penny had the most influence over Rosie, and influenced her so that she signed the consent forms she should never have signed.

Rosie was no longer Rosie. She lost part of herself forever. Her family was being destroyed by what had happened to her through treatment which didn't actually get rid of her voices in the way it was meant to at all – but ended up producing another harsher voice, which destroyed any hope she might have once had. The hope of becoming a whole person was forever lost, due to the side effects of the E.C.T.

The psychiatrist had a deep dark secret concerning the treatment. One of the major side effects of E.C.T was significant memory loss. Now most psychiatrists seem to be under the impression, however ill-informed they are that it is only a very small amount of memory that gets affected. But in actual fact, instead of just blotting out unwanted parts of a person's mind, such as blocking the voices out so that they are no longer heard, what actually happens in the terrifying reality is that whole sections of a person's mind are eventually blotted out. The secret case of memory loss in the worst case the psychiatrist had seen in a patient was the fact that they could no longer remember anything at all about what had happened to them in their childhood.

20th Century medicine: The days of enlightenment. No longer the dark ages. One would hope that at the very least the patients could change their minds about having the treatment if they so wished, but no. Dozens of young teenage girls had sat in that waiting room, hearing the floorboards creaking below, petrified – wanting to say no, but knowing they were the next ones to walk into the lion's den. There they would face the lion and be completely consumed by it. No hope, no going forward to face it, to run away from it, and no turning back.

Rosie was hopeful about this treatment, which the doctors had told her was the only answer to her problems. They were quite simply just running out of options, because Rosie wouldn't cooperate. Penny was the only member of staff who seemed to be able to manage to convince her that she needed help at all. But she refused to admit to anyone, her family, or even herself that there was a problem. She didn't feel that she needed to have any treatment. Medicine taking was hardly convenient. It was really a total intrusion on her everyday life. She found it intimidating to be bound to a routine; she didn't need to have her life running like clockwork, based on appointments, visits to the psychiatrist, and visits from the social workers who were forever plaguing her when she didn't want to communicate with anybody except her voices.

Her voices were her only friends. They kept her informed of what to do, what to say, who was safe and who was not. But she didn't entertain any idea that they might be false friends – that they'd give her false information, and false ideas. They convinced her to believe that everyone in her family was against her apart from her stepfather, David. David was so warm, caring, and confident, somebody that Rosie could go to for a kiss and a hug when she was feeling lonely. She couldn't cope with the atmosphere between her and her mother at all, which was continually fraught with tension. Melanie passed on to her daughter how worried she was feeling about the fact that she'd refuse to cooperate with anyone who was trying to help her. As far as Melanie was concerned though, she was always a failure, because her daughter had passed beyond the barriers of hope.

Melanie looked at the psychiatric ward as a place of respite for her family. But it was, in fact, anything but that. How could it be anything else, when Melanie should have realised that her daughter was in safekeeping, a place of safety, a haven of safety? She shouldn't need to be worrying any more, not now the staff had made Rosie their personal responsibility. But why was their family life completely disrupted by the anxiety that Rosie passed on to her relatives, even when she was being cared for by others? If Rosie had been a "good girl", been submissive, done exactly as she had been told by those people who, however Rosie saw them (and she always saw them as intruders), actually DID know better than she did, they knew what was best for her and after all, they WERE trained medical professionals.

If the situation on the ward had been any different, if Melanie hadn't seen things going on which shouldn't have been seen, or heard, by the next of kin, maybe she would have been able to deal with the mounting stress that she was already under through constantly worrying about Rosie. In any event, what would be the outcome of what might happen to Rosie? There was no way that Melanie was happy about leaving Rosie alone on the ward, with no family around her watching out for her, making sure what her needs really were.

Without strong family support, what might happen to anyone who found themselves isolated in that terrible situation? It is a wonder any of them lived through to the next day, actually. Melanie knew deep down in her heart that she'd done everything humanely possible to protect Rosie from what now seemed to be completely unavoidable. E.C.T spelled the end of their family life forever. Maybe the reason the family started falling apart was due to the devastating disappointment each one of them felt when the realisation that Rosie was now lost, completely beyond all hope. Penny had raised the family's hopes by promising that the E.C.T treatment would work without a doubt. They would find Rosie a completely changed person.

Indeed, she had changed. But it could hardly be called "changed for the better." When all the treatment had succeeded in doing would be to get the rest of the family into the psychiatrist's room more quickly.

David was proving to be just as impossible as his stepdaughter when it came to trying to persuade him that "yes" indeed there was a massive family crisis looming, and they all owed it to Rosie to make sure that it didn't happen the way that Melanie was petrified it would. However, Melanie couldn't understand why David was being so evasive about facing this together. It was as if he went into complete denial about what was going on between him and Melanie, who was already feeling that it was impossible to talk to her husband. He never had time. Busyness.

Busyness. Being busy was his one formula to escape from facing up to the truth about himself.

"Does he understand how trapped I am feeling? He can't do, but then I'm not even sure that he is aware of anybody else apart from himself, these days," thought Melanie.

Rosie was due to have another crisis, which was why Melanie became adamant that the family needed to get professional help, and fast. That is, if they weren't all too busy. "Too busy". That seemed to be the phrase that they used these days – too busy to think, too busy to listen, too busy to hear, too busy to notice and without a doubt, too busy to see inside of themselves.

Melanie desperately needed more time and space, even just to be able to tune into what was happening with her and David. But she couldn't get him to open up and talk to her, which was why she felt that he was somehow absent. There a lot of the time, but not there. Rosie was the one thing driving them apart from each other, and yet keeping them together through her troubles.

It was Rosie's voices tearing their family apart. Telling Rosie things, convincing her that everyone else was totally against her, when the truth was that they were actually not. The voices made her shut her mother out completely, and sent her running into David's warm, tender arms. Rosie was just a vulnerable little girl, who was completely deceived, completely naïve. She was too naïve to even notice the danger that she was getting herself into every time she turned to David for comfort and support. She argued, and argued that she was perfectly ok with the situation, she didn't feel used by him in any way at all, and it never occurred to her that what was actually happening between them was dreadfully wrong. Until they arranged for the whole family to go to see the therapist together and Penny could finally make Rosie understand that she really did need to get help.

Rosie's voices gave the game away. They let out the secret so Melanie heard loud and clear what was happening between her husband and daughter, his stepdaughter. She could see the relationship getting totally out of control, because she knew Rosie had the tendency to form completely unrealistic attachments and that she had no concept that anything wrong was being done to her, until he pushed her just that little bit too far over the edge.

The voices. Let's go back and try to hear what they are saying. It just may be the case that they have something really important to say to everyone, who might hear them, if they would only listen.

Melanie must have been sitting in the hospital canteen for a good two hours at least, by now. She still hadn't had the phone call she'd been waiting for the whole of that morning. So she found her sense of relief almost overwhelming when her phone did eventually ring. Where could Rosie have got to all this time? There were only so many places in the hospital she could possibly be. Melanie knew the voices must have been behind her disappearance. Finally, there was a voice on the other end of the mobile, not just a recorded message, and at least she wasn't just being put on hold.
"David, it's Rosie. I'm at the hospital. She's run off, and they can't find where she is." "I'm coming," said David.

David soon arrived on the scene to find his stepdaughter surrounded by a group of scary-looking psychiatric nurses, one of which was waving a needle in the air. "It's almost as if they are brandishing it like a switchblade." thought David. "They'll never get her to co-operate with them like this." So he went to see the ward sister. "Please let me have some time alone to talk to my stepdaughter. If you don't I'm afraid that I'm going to have no choice but to insist that this place is totally unsuitable for her to live in." said David.

"Sir, I'm afraid that we just can't allow her to come out of our sight, right now. The situation is much too serious. She could be a danger to herself, and a danger to other people. It's not safe to let her roam free in the community without adequate medical supervision, quite apart from the fact that she won't take her medication properly. She seems to think she's all right, once she comes out of the hospital, and stops taking it much too soon. As far as we can see, she has two options, both of which mean that she absolutely definitely needs to stay here for a great deal longer than she is willing to. She also needs the support from every single member of her family. Now this idea will definitely need everyone to agree to participate." With that, the ward sister turned to Melanie. "Do you think you and your husband would have any objections to all going to see the psychiatrist together?" Melanie didn't really know how to respond. It put her in quite a predicament, especially as she was communicating with David less and less.

"I think you will need to speak to David alone about this" she told Penny. "All I want is the best help available to Rosie, and I am sure that he must feel the same way. Why don't you speak to him and Rosie together, because I think you will get a better response from him if you do. I don't seem able to get anything out of him these days. She'll talk to him, I know she will. But whether she'll be willing to talk with more than one person around is anybody's guess, the way she's feeling at the moment" replied Melanie.

She still hadn't had that phone call from the police – and she was beginning to feel even more panicky – but she knew that the only thing that would make her feel any better would be if David turned up. Thankfully, she didn't have to wait long. He managed to arrive on the ward half an hour later – which meant Melanie was able to heave a sigh of relief. She hadn't any idea that she was feeling so upset and anxious, without David's support around. But David's reaction to Melanie wasn't the one that she was expecting from him. She'd hoped and prayed that he would be his old, caring and supportive self, when it came to Rosie, but she had never seen him so angry. "What's the matter?" she asked, tentatively.

"Why do you have to bother me at work?" He grunted. "You knew that I couldn't get away any sooner. I want to see Rosie. Where is she?"

"She's not here, David."

"I hold you totally responsible, especially if anything happens to her." He exploded with rage.

Distraught, by now, Melanie began to cry. Tears rolled down her cheeks. It was such a good thing that Penny was a good listener and really managed to connect with her patients. She connected with them much more than any of the other staff had done on previous occasions. Melanie had felt so guilty about the frequent visits to the hospital that she didn't even feel able to pick up the phone and call 999 for help without feeling as if it was all a total waste of time. Perhaps the doctors would be right about the E.C.T blocking out the voices. But what Melanie hadn't bargained for was that the voices were also blocking out everything else as well, so that her daughter was put in the position of being somebody she no longer knew, Rosie was becoming a total stranger.

CLAUDE DEBUSSY: GARDENS IN THE RAIN

Jolts of electricity. Rosie thought that was what was meant by E.C.T. She didn't even want to have the treatment. She felt as if she were being treated like somebody, maybe one of those 'mad' Victorian women who needed to be locked away in a Victorian asylum, to be put on public view and shown off for the amusement of the gentry. Was this really the 21st century? From the way she was being forced into signing forms for treatment, and the way the staff talked down to her all the time, as if she were two years old, not a young woman, she was absolutely sure that the staff had had no proper training in how to communicate with their patients and their families. For a start, a patient's parents were already upset by anything that they might have had to go through as a result of any crisis that had bought them into a situation of accepting help from the hospital in the first place.

Rosie knew Melanie was depressed. She also suspected that Melanie blamed her for everything else that was going wrong in the family, including the break-up of Melanie's relationship with David. Actually, Rosie did feel guilty for having such a dreadful secret to hide. She thought the world of her stepfather. It was him that she clung to for emotional strength and support, because somehow his strength helped to push the strength of her voices backwards so that they gradually faded, and the stronger feelings started to emerge from David's warmth – the warmth of the physical closeness and contact.

Rosie was naïve. She didn't know she was being sexually abused. She felt safe and protected, even though this had started a long time ago, when she was desperately under-age. She'd carried this guilty secret around with her for at least two years now. But she couldn't bear the atmosphere of the stress and mounting tension in the family. However, because of the disintegrating conversations between Melanie and David, Rosie was fully aware that Melanie and David no longer slept together, because she was the one who was sleeping with David on a regular basis. No wonder Melanie felt communication between family members was totally disintegrating. But what Melanie had no idea about at all was the fact that she was being frequently deceived by the daughter. She thought she could completely trust her. Melanie blamed herself for absolutely everything. She could trust David, because he loved her.

As Rosie sat in the waiting room, biding her time to go into the lion's den, she felt a sense of optimism. A glimmer of hope, that she would never again be plagued by those piercing voices, which would be silenced forever after this afternoon.

She wanted to forget – so much. There was so much she wanted to block in her mind, so much which was too difficult to deal with.

"It's time now, dear" said Penny, leading her gently by the arm.

Time for what? Did Rosie have a clue about what was going to happen to her?

The next three-quarters of an hour would change not just her life but also the lives of her entire family. She hadn't been given all the facts. They were supposed to tell her all the implications of the treatment that she'd signed for when she put her pen across the dotted line, but she failed to see the small print in between the lines. The nurses should have made sure she had access to information about the E.C.T, but they were fearful that she'd refuse to have it done, that there would be too much confrontation. They were the ones who were scared of confrontation.

There is nothing wrong with speaking out against the authorities, the powers-that be, the hierarchies. The ones who have the powers the patients should have, they should have the power to be the great "I AM", not the staff. It's all about them, after all. So, what are the staff scared of?

The real crux of the matter might be, in actual fact, that it's the staff that have something to hide, not the patients. So why is it easier for staff to deal with patients walking around the wards looking like zombies? Patients who are so unstimulated for whom the wards start to look little better than the insides of the gas chambers of a nazi concentration camp? The staff seem scared of patients becoming "too excited". Perhaps this is really because they are fearful of the "mad" voice, which in their opinion, needs to be dampened down as much as possible. It seems fitting that the psychiatric wards are often housed in big old Victorian buildings, and the patients treated little better than the madwoman locked away, out of society's reach, forgotten. The patients are best forgotten. They are unacceptable to modern day society. Any time spent on the wards result in patients forgetting their true identity.

FORGETTING TRUE IDENTITY, THE UNREAD BLUE-PRINT OF THE DREADED E.C.T. AND THE VISIT TO THE LION'S DEN

When Rosie's treatment had finished, she found that she could remember nothing. Not even being admitted onto the ward, or where she was. She had difficulty remembering the day of the week, or what time of day it was. She couldn't even remember who Melanie and David were. Melanie had been given plenty of previous warning about the memory-loss, but was reassured that the memory would return to its full capacity, given time.

That was the great-unanswered question now though. They would just have to "wait and see". They were all facing a whole long week's wait, at least to see if there were any detrimental side effects. What they couldn't understand is that they felt experimented on, like guinea pigs. Surely it was fairer that the nurses already knew what the side effects would be, before being allowed to administer treatment to vulnerable people in the first place. Something wasn't right. Side effects. Ignorance is bliss. Something Melanie could never forget after this. The only thing Melanie could do now was to sit by her sleeping daughter, and hope that she would be able to remember something when she woke up. That was the best that she could hope for.

Melanie had decided to take a brief break from sitting by Rosie's bed, keeping watch. She decided to go for a walk around the hospital grounds. It was spring now, and the banks were filled with rows and rows of golden daffodils. Walking always did the trick when it came to Melanie handling her anxiety levels. There was no sign of any life yet, as Rosie showed no signs of waking up. Melanie decided to take a chance and make the most of the opportunity to unwind.

Ten minutes later, Rosie opened her eyes. She couldn't even remember her own name, or where she was, but she knew she had been dreaming, vividly. She could remember her dream right down to the very last detail. The picture she had seen in her mind's eye during the period of being semi-conscious, but asleep and half awake, gradually drifting in and out of the two states of conscious. The images were incredibly vivid. She could remember it so clearly, that she could give a completely accurate description of the images, as they came sharply into focus, even when she was conscious of the fact that she was becoming more fully aware.

Rosie could see a huge tree. At first, all she could make out were lots of branches, of different sizes and shapes, thick branches and thin branches, but the picture that stuck in her mind the most, was one of the big flowers at the end of every branch. Beautiful flowers, with amazingly pretty petals, masses of them. The petals were closed up, as if they were enormous buds that hadn't started opening, yet. They were roughly the same shape and size as tulips. Rosie could make out different colours in the mainly white petals, but the petals were also half- coloured in streaks of light pink. She couldn't remember the name of the tree to begin with. But soon, the name "Magnolia" came into a much sharper focus. Why was she thinking about a Magnolia tree? In what way might it have been significant in her life? She couldn't begin to place where.
There seemed to be no clues.

Struggling desperately to remember the tree's location, Rosie's mind drew a blank, then went into the blackness of total oblivion, Rosie drifted back into her unconscious state, which was the most comfortable one she could deal with, right now.

The implications of what she'd experienced had not really registered their true impact on her yet. She was only conscious of a dark void, as if it were part of the eternal abyss. The only way she could switch off from the feeling of travelling down a deep tunnel, with a sense of nothingness all the way down it, to the very bottom, was to shut her eyes and return to a state of being half awake, and half asleep. She wasn't certain what state she was in.

The image of the colourful petals gradually became more sharply focused. The tree re-emerged, but its reflection now included freshly cut green grass. As Rosie began to regain consciousness, she wondered and wondered in bewilderment. Why the Magnolia tree was significant in her life? As her thoughts gradually resurfaced, she found herself questioning: "Why is the tree so symbolic in some way? Does it belong somewhere special in my life? Is it part of my present, or maybe symbolic of my future in some way, even?" But in spite of all her continuing thoughts, whirling around in her head, she never once looked back on her childhood. She couldn't go there, down that pathway of her mind. She felt strange on the inside. Something had significantly changed. Part of her personality had gone, for good. Lost for eternity.

But the Magnolia tree remained.

Rosie struggled to make sense of why the tree might be important to her. She felt she was on the inside of something, looking out. Each time she had experienced that feeling, she was looking out of a glass window, and beyond the window she could see the beautiful tree outside in the garden. The picture was unclear because of the raindrops appearing on the panes of glass. Suddenly the raindrops started falling faster, faster and faster, pattering against the glass preventing Rosie from seeing the tree at all..

As the mistiness from her brain began to clear, the flowers came more sharply into focus, so they became much more precise and defined, "That's a Magnolia tree" was the first thought Rosie was able to voice as she regained consciousness. She could see shadows of three people standing by her bedside. They were just shadows. She couldn't really make out who the shapes were at all, except for David. The voices knew him of old. Rosie stated speaking loudly in a voice that wasn't hers.
"DAVID .... David.... David........." Rosie's voices echoed around the room. Then:
"DON'T TOUCH ME! Don't touch me... Don't touch me. No! No! No! ...."
With that, the nurses grabbed David and escorted him out of the room. Their patient had now become "Too excited."

PART 2
THE COLOUR WHEEL. The Sketch of The Artist
Claude Monet: The Poppy Field

The portrait was painted by each stroke of the brush, producing different colours, the shape, form and style all merged together .The artist also had a need to function on his own, painting in the countryside, walking past the blazing red poppy field to find a place near the golden hay fields where he could place his easel and paint the delicate petals of the poppies.

Each stroke of his brush delicately defined the beauty of each individual petal, light red, dark red, the different shades merging the colours together to make a whole. The artist had the opportunity of reading into the depths of the human soul, understanding empathy, the ability to just be there and not impose upon a person's private space, so that person could create their own art form, so they could reach their own potential, and depths of self-understanding.

MAKING SHADES OF GREY
Confusion and Denial

The hospital room suddenly seemed to be filled with utter confusion. Rosie had drifted back into her unconscious state, which was just as well for her, as it happened, because she had no idea of the absolute chaos she had caused over the last few minutes. Now the nurses had another unconscious person to deal with in the room. Melanie had collapsed with shock.

Penny was kneeling at her side, helping her to have a glass of water as soon as she showed signs that she was coming round. Melanie looked dreadful. The emotional turmoil of the last few months, what with everything going wrong with Rosie, and now it seemed that she could no longer rely on her main support system in the way that she'd grown so used to doing over the last few years, meant that Melanie's whole world had been torn apart by the shocking revelations that had been revealed by the family's biggest enemy: The voices. They shouldn't even be there, any longer. They had no right to be there after the E.C.T. The E.C.T was supposed to silence them, not make them stronger. Melanie's hopes and dreams of a normal family life had been dashed, all in a matter of ten minutes.

The last ten minutes had totally transformed their family life. Destroyed everything Melanie had ever believed in, everything she had fought for.

She had fought so hard on her daughter's behalf, even though the health care authorities had told her time and time again that she was wasting her time. She'd done everything to provide each member of her family with loving care, and support, and a comfortable family home, she'd devoted her entire life to it. Suddenly, her cosy, middle-class life, her suburbia, was shattered in an instant. How could over twenty-five years of one's entire life be lost completely in just ten minutes? Life was so fragile. One never knew what lay around the corner. Depression made it difficult to appreciate what one really had. Depression robbed not just one person of their joy, and hope, but everyone around them. Melanie woke up to the fact that she had probably been just as depressed as Rosie had been.

Melanie's entire existence over the last few months had become so taken over by her daughter's illness that she'd had no time to even think about her own health, or her own needs. It was now evident that her body was starting to kick against the strain of the present circumstances; especially now Melanie had no props. She hadn't realised she'd always used David as a prop, ever since she'd known him, to cover up her own sense of inadequacy. So what were the possibilities now? What would be in store for her future? Melanie couldn't think straight to see any sort of a pathway or that there might be room for tremendous freedom and personal growth, if she had to stand-alone.

All she could think about was the betrayal by her daughter and her husband. The thought of both of them, together, left her reeling, feeling too physically sick to want to eat properly for days on end. The only thought that Melanie had now was to get David out of her life for good. There was no room in their relationship for a third party. Some women might be able to put up with that, just to keep their husbands for as long as possible, but not Melanie. Melanie faced tough choices. She wondered how on earth she would be strong enough, or would find the strength from inside herself. Did she have strength there that she'd never seen until now? Did she avoid having to look on the inside for a long time, because it was too challenging, and she didn't want to be bothered to change, because she was too comfortable with her cosy, middle-class suburbia existence? So that it was turning into some kind of fantasy world?

It had never occurred to Melanie that she might be sick herself; so much of her time and energy had been spent focusing on her daughter's problems. Perhaps the fact that she was so engrossed in trying to make life run more smoothly for the others in her family had become part of one great denial of truth.

THE STARK TRUTH

Melanie WAS mentally ill herself. Something she couldn't even begin to accept, or understand. Why was this happening to her, and her family? *How could over twenty-five years of one's life be lost completely in five seconds?* Melanie was slowly waking up to the fact that she had probably been just as depressed as Rosie had always been. Melanie's entire existence over the last few years had become so taken over by her daughter's illness that she'd had no time to even think about her own health, or her own needs. It was now evident that her body was beginning to kick against the strain of the current circumstances, especially as Melanie now had no props.

Melanie wondered how on earth she'd be strong enough, to find the strength, but perhaps she'd never seen before now. Because she'd avoided having to look on the inside for a long time, because it was too challenging, and she didn't want to be bothered to change, because she was too comfortable with the cosy, middle-class existence that now seemed as if it were turning into some kind of fantasy world. *It had never occurred to Melanie that she might be sick herself, so much of her time and energy had been spent on sorting out her daughter's problems. Perhaps the fact that she was so engrossed in trying to make life run more smoothly for the other people in her family had become part of one great denial of truth. Stark truth. The stark truth stung, painfully. Melanie WAS mentally ill herself. Something she couldn't accept or even begin to understand. Why was this happening to her?* If she was ill herself, why couldn't she accept it? Maybe it was because of the label already given to her family by the mental health services. Their numbers were already on a computer system. Numbers without a name. Perhaps that was why the psychiatric services seemed so keen on the idea of giving their psychiatric patients a "label". The title for a psychiatric ward should be: "DIAGNOSE THIS! THE REALITY OF LIVING WITH A PSHYCHIATRIC DIAGNOSIS"

Melanie couldn't accept the label 'nutter' that accompanied most of the patients she had come into contact with. She wasn't a 'nutter'. So why did this have to happen to her and her family? Was it some kind of punishment for a past life? "I'm the one holding everything together, being everyone else's stability, so how come I am now one of the 'mad' people?" she agonised, not realising that she was displaying classic symptoms of denial, a normal response from anyone when they first hear what their problem was. They feel shame for being told they are 'mad'. The treatments help nothing. Dampening the mad voice. Telling patients they are "too excited", just by being put into normal, stimulating environments suddenly becomes too much for them to cope with. Drugging innocent people up to their eyeballs should be treated as a major criminal offence, so why is it suddenly acceptable for the staff to treat people in such a barbaric manner? Hitler never got away with gassing millions of Jews during the Holocaust; a psychiatric ward is not a ghetto. The psychiatrist is not Adolf Hitler; neither are their nursing staff the Nazis.

Melanie felt deep shame as it dawned on her that she'd been depressed for a long time. She couldn't voice the way she felt for the shame and embarrassment that was making her reluctant to talk about it openly. But, if she didn't come clean soon, then there was a greater danger that the anger would be buried deeply inside, and that it would become introverted anger, turning into an even angrier depression.

Melanie felt guilty about David, about not knowing what was going on between him and Rosie. She now knew the only option she had was to force David to leave the family home. So she arranged with Penny to help remove all of his belongings from their house, and had all the locks changed. David was now the one left out in the cold.

Society doesn't make it any easier for new psychiatric patients because of the intolerance of mental health within the community, and even in the hospitals themselves. Melanie wondered how many real friends she'd still have, once this got out. She also found herself filled with sympathy for Rosie. What had Rosie been going through, all this time? Melanie had only just discovered there was something wrong, and Rosie had had to grow up within the constraints of being "labelled." No wonder her teenage years had now proven to be so turbulent. It is bad enough, even as a teenager with a normal life and stable background struggling, sometimes with devastating consequences. Suddenly, Melanie was filled with a deep sense of respect and admiration for her daughter, with this new, fresh understanding.

Hoping Rosie would regain consciousness, perhaps there would be a chance to remould their relationship on a fresh footing. Melanie felt that she had wronged her daughter terribly. But what would happen when she finally woke up? Would Melanie ever have the chance to make it up to her daughter that she now so longed for? Would Rosie be the same, or be a person that none of them knew? What would she be like, without her voices? It must be odd, being stripped completely bare of something that had been part of her for as long as any of them could remember.

Still, Rosie showed no signs of life. The hours passed. Day turned into night. Night turned into yet another day.

Melanie was no closer to accepting the harsh truth about herself and her family, or what had been tearing her family apart all this time. Her feelings were changing. She suddenly changed from being sympathetic and understanding into complete dread. The reality of what had actually happened between Rosie and David, the two people who were most precious to her. She felt totally devastated. Things were never going to be the same again.

RUBY RED

Penny had suggested to Melanie that she should go home to rest. There seemed to be little point in waiting at Rosie's bedside indefinitely, not whilst it was apparently going to be a considerably long time before she regained consciousness. Penny was worried about Melanie. She looked totally warn out and exhausted. Penny's warm, caring nature won Melanie over, every single time. Melanie agreed to go home to spend the afternoon catching up on all the sleep she'd missed out on since her daughter was admitted onto the psychiatric ward. Penny promised to let Melanie know what was happening to Rosie, as soon as there were any changes. Melanie went home, because she trusted Penny.

But what she hadn't ever imagined was that Rosie was going to end up in a deep crisis before her return. The Accident and Emergency Department at the hospital was always extra busy on a Saturday night. The trolleys were always filled with people, waiting to see the doctors specialists, and psychiatrists. On that particular Saturday evening, every single side-room and all the cubicles were filled. The ward was jampacked full of patients, and the staff were pushed to their limits because they were short staffed.

As if this wasn't enough for them to handle, without extraordinary activity going on – which would have been the last thing on their minds. It was hard enough dealing with simple, routine medical matters with the queues of people waiting for at least five hours before even beginning to diminish.

Two psychiatric patients on the run, not having been spotted by the staff on their own ward, was not something the A and E staff had even thought they might end up having to deal with that night, much less the fact that the situation was doomed to end in a full-scale tragedy.

At about four o'clock that afternoon, Rosie finally woke up, feeling much more like her normal self again. She still couldn't remember anything very well, but maybe this would improve gradually, as the side effects of being so heavily sedated wore off. When Rosie finally came around, she realised with shock, that she was alone. Penny was nowhere to be seen, Melanie wasn't there, and neither was David. Rosie felt very alone when she realised that there wasn't one single member of her family around. Rosie decided that she'd had enough of being in bed all this time, so decided to go for a walk. She hadn't realised that she'd feel quite so unsteady, when she finally got onto her feet. She had to hold onto the bed, and was thankful when she first started walking. She managed to make it to the main part of the ward. She was still petrified of the other patients in there. The patients didn't look like real people. They were behaving extremely oddly. Most of them seemed to be in a dreamlike world. Rosie knew instinctively that this was because of having to use psychiatric medication on a long-term basis.

There was one patient there, who seemed more alert than the others. He surveyed her, curiously. Rosie felt uncomfortable as he looked her up and down, it made her extremely nervous. "Your hair is so beautiful," he told her. Rosie had long, raven black hair, and blue eyes. She was tall and thin,

"Hello. My name is Rosie, what's yours?" she asked, tentatively.

"Jamie McBride" He answered in a thick Scottish accent. "Are you lost?"

"No, but I want to get out of here for a while, it is driving me nuts. I need some fresh air" Rosie replied.

"Let's go for a walk," Jamie suggested. Rosie nodded. There were no members of staff in sight, as they managed to escape from the ward, unnoticed by anyone. This should never have happened, because Rosie had been sectioned under 24 hour scrutiny, because she was a danger to herself, and now it was also questionable as to whether she would now put others at risk should she be feeling aggressive enough. Trained psychiatric staff were concerned about her lashing out. They treat patients in a completely inhumane way, believing they are being deliberately violent. This just goes to show how dangerous and inappropriate it is to ever make assumptions when it comes to other people.

Don't psychiatric nursing staff ever stop to wonder what it is like to hear voices, or have to cope with manic depression, with life treating you a bit like a yo-yo.?

Sometimes it seems that staff are so sadly lacking the basic counselling and empathy skills. If they only TALKED to each patient, say for thirty minutes, to find out what's REALLY happening to them, they would save the patient and their family from a great deal of unnecessary suffering and heartache, and maybe even manage to save lives before it's too late. The nurses compound the problems with the fear factor and even cause stigma themselves. There does seem to be some kind of a power struggle going on between staff and patients.

The dampening down of the 'mad' voice suggests that the staff have something they're hiding, but being forced to keep quiet about it is probably the least helpful thing that can possibly happen to a person who has just been diagnosed with a mental illness. There is little wonder then, that fellow-sufferers often find solace in each other, because their experiences of their world and individual dealings with illness can mean a lot of common bonding.

Rosie and Jamie had been missing for two hours before the staff noticed they'd gone. It wasn't even the staff on the psychiatric ward that noticed they'd gone missing either. Rosie and Jamie were sitting on a bench in the hospital grounds, overlooking the banks filled with the yellow, golden daffodils, that Melanie had appreciated so much. Rosie was starting to feel weak again. Jamie leant forward, putting his arms around her, when he discovered that she was shaking, trembling all over. She shut her eyes, feeling nauseous and dizzy. "Come on, you'll be fine, soon" Jamie told her. "It's great to get out of there, isn't it?"

"Sure. But I don't feel well at all. Maybe we should head back," said Rosie.

"Not yet" Jamie said. "There's something I want to do, first."

"Oh?" enquired Rosie

Jamie started to stroke Rosie's long black hair.

"What the hell do you think you're doing?" Rosie said trying to pull away from him, but he was much stronger than she was.

"It'll be fine. Trust me"

He took her by the hand, and led her to a secluded spot where no one would be able to find them. Rosie wasn't comfortable. This man was a total stranger. "I don't want this," she told him.

"Why did you come with me, then?" he said, starting to lose his temper.

"I just wanted a walk". Rosie was now starting to panic, as it began to dawn on her that this was not what he had had in mind at all. Suddenly his hands were wandering all over her body. He started squeezing and fondling her breasts, and touching her in intimate places. Rosie knew that she'd be unable to stop, because it always made her feel helpless whenever anybody touched her there, in that way. "PLEASE stop now, PLEASE." she began pleading with him. "NO - STOP! You're HURTING me." Tears now started falling down Rosie's cheeks as she realised she could not escape the crushing weight of this big man's body, pushing harder and harder against her own weak, frail feminine form. She was feeling sicker and sicker as she waited for the inevitable encounter with the intimate part of the male anatomy. She could feel it was becoming harder and harder and soon he was thrusting in and out of her, taking full advantage of being stronger than she was. The male sex IS the stronger sex. Women are the 'weaker' ones, supposedly. Jamie began to exert every part of his male authority over her Rosie so that she became completely intimidated.

Rosie was being raped.

So this is what it felt like. It was so different with David. David was gentle, warm and sweet. How could it be wrong? It couldn't be the same when she wanted David as badly as he wanted her. It didn't even occur to her that it was wrong because she was under age, and that he was married to her mother.

Rosie started to push Jamie off, turning on her heels she ran. Jamie ran after her, but Rosie knew how to get back to the ward. The hospital was so confusing with its long corridors. She ran to the nearest ward, Jamie chasing her in hot pursuit.

The nursing staff DID notice them. Rosie's voices were calling her all the while, "Rosie, Rosie, Rosie, Rosie..." above the chaos, making Rosie panic into taking flight. The nursing staff were alerted by the fact that there were two patients from the psychiatric ward on the run, and raised the alarm. They also dialled 999, as Jamie was well known for being a violent patient, especially around women. But the patients were unable to stop

running. Rosie was running from Jamie. Jamie was running from his past, present and future. He managed to grab Rosie, and put his hand over her mouth to stifle her screams, which were becoming louder and louder. What Jamie hadn't realised is that there were policemen everywhere now.

Jamie decided on the spur of the moment, that it was time to leave Rosie to it, and make his escape. Rosie had decided to co-operate for once, not before time, either. Rosie could never believe that any of the staff were acting in her best interests. She couldn't even understand that going into hospital was in her best interests either. Everything and everyone was totally against her. But she needed to feel safe. If she couldn't feel safe in hospital, where on earth could she be safe? Nowhere is safe, and no one is safe, not on a psychiatric ward when you have a mental illness.

Jamie took to his heels and ran. He kept running, running, running and running. He didn't look where he was going. He didn't know where this was leading to. He found a door, pushed it open, he was facing lots and lots of flights of stairs, he ran up one, then another and another and another, until he'd reached the top. The top was on the 8th floor up. The police followed in hot pursuit. As Jamie came out of the corridor, the police were catching up with him. Outside the lift was a huge glass window. Jamie was out of breath. He stopped, panting for air, not realising the window was right behind him. He backed away from the police, as far away as he could possibly go.

SMASH! Cracked glass smashed to smithereens scattered all over the place, falling outside as well as inside. Jamie lost his footing, falling headfirst from the 6th floor window. There was a mighty thud. His body lay on the ground outside. Pools of blood were forming everywhere.

Rosie had always known the voices would lead her to tragedy one day. Today was THE day. THIS was it. This had to be the ultimate tragedy.

MISTY BLUE

Rosie still felt totally confused and out of sorts. The one thing she felt compelled to do was escape. She had to run, but this had to be planned. Her voices were telling her to plan a massive escape from the army, police and the navy, who were all planning to go into the first stages of the battle of World War III. It was up to Rosie to plan a complicated escape route from the concentration camp.

Her mind felt totally disorientated. Drugged up to the eyeballs, looking and feeling like a Jew emerging from a gas chamber, Rosie felt invincible. She was the one who was going to win this battle. Not realising the battle was in her mind. She'd lost all contact with reality. She had no idea what day it was, what time of day it was, or even where she was. Struggling, she tried to lay her master escape plan, but her mind wasn't functioning enough to work out where she'd head for without any help with living arrangements. She couldn't remember how to use a phone. She hated using one, as it was when she didn't feel very well, in any case. Was her best bet to make a run for it, or to enlist the help of a secret agent? What about the timing of her action plan? There wasn't enough time to find a secret agent to help the spies were all over the place. No, maybe Rosie's best bet would be to make a run for her freedom and liberty completely unaided. But perhaps if she had a secret agent, it would help her to find a way through the clouded misty blue. She was petrified that the spies and traitors would prevent her from finding her liberty, try to restore her back to sanity.

But was she really insane? Why did she feel invincible, capable of anything? She was capable of mapping out "The Great Escape" all by herself. She didn't need a secret agent. She didn't need a passport, either. She had the help of the army. Maybe she could even fly herself. Maybe, if she tried climbing to the top of the building and onto the roof, once she'd jumped off, she felt as if she'd be able to fly. The wind would carry her. The wind was her strength. The secret agent would hamper her progress. She'd need to send messages to the army in Morse code, SOS messages, so that she'd be on her way. She'd have to escape from Adolf Hitler. They had made an appointment for her to go to see him, but she was scared that she'd end up being shot, once she got into that room alone with him. She looked around at the rest of the Jews waiting to go into the gas chambers. What use was going in there possible going to be to them? What answers to the humanitarian crisis did Adolf Hitler possibly have to offer anyone? She couldn't understand why everyone thought he had the answers. Surely the answers came from inside the soul. Rosie found herself fighting endless battles within her inner self. She felt she was going through World War III. Maybe if she did go in there and talk to Adolf Hitler he'd have the answers to her misery, maybe it would be easier for everyone if he just shot her anyway. She couldn't even bear the idea of revealing all her secrets to someone she barely knew. How could talking to a total stranger for twenty minutes possibly provide the answers to a whole lifetime of misery and heartache? But here was all her family, trying to insist that she walked into the room whether she wanted to go in there or not. They, it seemed, knew what was best for her. They had already decided that it was best for Rosie to come right out into the open with everything that she kept hidden from the whole of the rest of the world. Rosie knew she'd end up losing her entire family, once the real truth was out. Could she live with herself? She was the one who'd have to lice with herself for the rest of her life, knowing she'd broken up the relationship between her mum and step dad. Even though she felt so terribly torn between loyalties to Melanie, whom she still knew had devoted her entire life to putting her needs first, she wasn't able to let go of how she felt about David. The episode with Jamie McBride had showed her what her real feelings for her step dad were. She loved him. She sincerely believed that the love they shared couldn't possibly be wrong. She felt so much older than her fourteen years. She'd felt as if she'd been carrying the weight of the whole world on her young shoulders. People had always told her that she looked more like an eighteen year old than a fourteen year old. Being raped had completely confused Rosie's moral judgment. It almost seemed as if she'd never had any conscience. She was old enough to know it was right to have a sexual relationship with somebody who ought to have known better, and if he'd really cared anything for Rosie, would have stopped it, long before it had started. David was the one who seemed to be the first to blame her, but then, he was a man, with sexual needs. Rationality didn't come into it. David's arms were holding her, warm and close, she just felt as if she were melting into them. The cold shock and violence of being raped by a stranger was what she'd always understood rape to be.

They were all sitting in the room, facing Adolf Hitler, who was now asking Rosie streams of endless questions. Rosie couldn't quite remember the answers to any of them. She'd had her first flashback of the Magnolia tree when she'd regained consciousness, but now Adolf Hitler was interrogating her, probing her, trying to trip her up. Somehow, what she'd experienced might be some kind of punishment for a past life, but she couldn't even understand her present life, and it now seemed that there was a missing factor. She could only feel the pain from the perspective of her adult self. The child inside her had become lost. It needed to be found, but she couldn't trust Adolf Hitler to be the person to help her find her past. The person she trusted was David. He was the only person in the world who could make her feel loved. Now her child had disappeared to God knows where, she couldn't even connect to the part of herself that could give and receive love any more. David was her only hope, but just the simple act of being together meant that both of them ended up with so much more to lose.

How could Rosie cope in life without all the help and support that she'd received from Melanie? The realisation of how much time Melanie had devoted to her was only just beginning to dawn on Rosie. But her need for David was far greater than the knowledge of the wrong they were both doing by deceiving Melanie.

In comparison to how much she needed David, even this didn't matter to Rosie, even though she quickly realised that her relationship with her mother would never be able to be the same again. Rosie knew she had caused her deep sense of loss herself, by her own selfish actions. Even though she'd been so certain that Melanie would continue to be there for her, because of the completely selfless devoted way that she'd cared for Rosie, much more so than being concerned in any way at all about her own needs. Rosie knew that she had lost Melanie's trust entirely; that she would have lost part of herself, her true sense of identity seemed to be blocked off forever.

Although the E.C.T had already done much of the donkey-work, being deceitful was guaranteed to finish the job off completely. The E.C.T had robbed Rosie of any feelings of warmth, being able to give or receive it. Her relationship with David now proved itself to be the only outlet for her to be able to create warmth and love and now there was the constant threat of having somebody constantly watching over her. Rosie felt unable to connect to her feelings, or experience and express emotion. The fear that she had felt during the episode with Jamie McBride was something that was real enough, though she could have been mistaken for misunderstanding the definition of the word rape. She'd always understood it to be what had happened between her and Jamie. It was the rest of her that responded to giving and receiving warmth and love that had become lost and been totally destroyed in one afternoon.

At least guinea pigs had the choice of not realising what was happening to them when they were being experimented on. This was from a human perspective, though, not from that of the guinea pig, who's to say whether a guinea pig or any other animal come to that, is capable of feeling anything remotely human? Maybe they wouldn't be able to experience emotional reactions in the way that we humans understand them to be. Probably, the human race has got their interpretation of what love is completely wrong. Most folk think that it is some kind of idealized fantasy world of bubbly emotions, but never manage to find a true experience of real love in an entire lifetime. They get so busy looking for an idealised imaginary version of what they have grown up expecting it to be, that the real thing, if it ever emerges in life, stands a strong chance of passing one by like a ship in the night. There are so many facets of love, not least the love experienced in the close context of family. Love from other people is like a precious jewel, there, in an instant, if one doesn't grab it with both hands then it is gone, disappeared forever, like the moonlight disappearing behind the cotton-wool clouds. Rosie was desperate to love both of her parents in the normal way, but she knew her love for David went far beyond that. She was forced into an impossible decision of having to choose between her parents. Whichever choice she made, she'd end up losing one, or both of them. Rosie longed not to have to make such a choice at all.

As things turned out though, the situation had already been taken out of hands entirely. David made the choice for her, through his own selfish actions, which actually did Rosie a favour. She found true love, but it wasn't coming from the source where she'd been looking for it, but from totally unexpected quarters.

LEMON AND LIME

Rosie panicked. She didn't know how she was going to cope with being back on the ward. All she knew was that she wanted to escape from the police, the hospital grounds were teeming with them. She didn't feel ready to face either of her parents as she managed to find her way back into the hospital without anybody noticing. Her voices were in complete control of her; she became somebody else, and was almost in a total trance like state. She didn't really take too much notice of her surroundings because the voices were drowning out the reality of everything else. She was in such a trance like state that no one could recognise her anyway, she was so sedated.

Meanwhile, Penny was comforting Melanie, who was slowly but surely breaking down completely. She'd started sobbing hysterically as soon as the accident had happened, and couldn't understand why Rosie had just taken off. What had happened had now meant it was even harder for her to be able to trust any of the nursing staff, not one, not even Penny. Somebody had to be held responsible for what had happened to her daughter during her family's absence. They hadn't been gone that long, after all. But none of the staff seemed to want to have any sort of responsibility for anything that had happened. This didn't help anything, and Melanie ended up feeling guilty for everything that Rosie was suffering.

The thing that had made Melanie feel the guiltiest was Rosie's episodes of self- harming. Melanie was made to feel a complete failure by the staff in charge. If she'd been a more competent mother, then her daughter wouldn't be in the situation of trying to destroy herself. But Melanie felt that it would have happened anyway, in spite of everything Melanie had tried to do to help Rosie. It certainly wasn't through lack of trying, the families were so often the ones who were blamed for any situation that the children found themselves in. It didn't seem to do much good, or make the slightest difference. Melanie had hardly had the chance to think about herself at all. Most family weekends seemed to be spent chasing too and from the Accident and Emergency Department after Rosie. Melanie was left wondering whether Rosie's problems had been caused by the lack of communication between the other members of her family. David could hardly be called a great talker, all that had happened between him and Melanie was either screaming and shouting, or a deathly silence that could cut the atmosphere with a knife. Rosie hadn't been encouraged to be open about her feelings enough. She'd had a close friend in school, a fellow self-harmer. Her body had been discovered swinging round and round, supported by a rope tied to the branches of a tree in the local park by a passer-by walking the dog.

That was when Rosie's voices seemed to become particularly harsh and prominent. It was also during that time that she had started to go to David for comfort and support. Melanie was in shock as she finally concluded that David was a liar, who was incapable of being remotely honest with her about anything. How could they continue to have any relationship at all, without being completely honest with each other? But now it was Melanie who needed support. She'd been spending every waking moment giving up everything to care for others. It had turned out to be completely futile. Everything she'd ever done for anybody in her family had been chucked right back in her face. She was sure of one thing, that she'd done absolutely nothing to deserve being treated so badly by the person she'd devoted her entire life to. Little wonder, then, that Melanie had felt that her life was now pointless. Her marriage had turned out to be based on a complete lie, her family wasn't normal in any sense of the word, but in any case, what did the word normal mean these days, as it was?

Funnily enough, she couldn't find it in her heart to blame Rosie for anything that had happened to her and David. Rosie still had some childhood innocence left. No, David was the one who was to blame. He was a liar, and a cheat. Melanie felt sick at the very thought of him touching her, every time she visualised him and Rosie together, she started retching. The E.C.T had completely confused Melanie. Why were Rosie's voices still there? Hadn't the treatment worked? Maybe Rosie had got so scared and confused by the treatment that this had caused her to run away. Maybe she couldn't function properly, and now couldn't recognise any of her family at all. But why had Rosie's personality changed so dramatically? Melanie knew that Rosie had sometimes been confused by her voices, but nothing like this had ever happened in the past. If only Rosie could have been able to talk to them, now she was probably petrified that she was going to be arrested, the hospital was teeming with police.

Melanie wasn't at all surprised that her daughter was nowhere to be seen. However, this didn't stop Melanie from being worried and concerned that her daughter might try to run away. This was something that she had always done in the past, when the going got rough. Melanie was doubly scared of it now though, because it meant that Rosie wouldn't remember to take her medication. She had been acting so oddly, ever since she'd been admitted onto the ward. But it had to be her voices plaguing and torturing the poor girl, until she had reached the stage of begging them for mercy. Melanie felt hopeless, and helpless in this situation. She didn't feel able to trust Penny any more, had they fully understood everything that had been presented to them on the consent form? The thing was so full of technical jargon, which they didn't really know the full meaning of. Maybe they hadn't been given the correct information at all, actually this seemed to be totally unfair to Rosie, she had always felt this had caused major problems to people with mental health problems. They were so often treated as dumb idiots, people trying to organise things from a stranger's point of view, on the outside of the situation, knowing nothing about the background and just assumed that they were not very intelligent, and therefore unable to think for themselves. This was highlighted by the fact the staff didn't feel it was particularly necessary to give their patients all the necessary information, before signing the complicated consent forms that they were expected to sign. Presumably the staff had reached that conclusion because of the outside appearance of a patient who has been very heavily sedated. They jump to the conclusions that the patient is either slow, or thick, and unable to think clearly for himself because of his illness, or psychosis. There isn't enough information about side effects of drugs, not even for the staff.

Melanie knew that Rosie had responded to the E.C.T. treatment by becoming disorientated, and had taken flight because that was her only alternative. Taking flight from being kept a prisoner, like a caged bird, ready to fly. The hospital was such a constrictive place. Melanie had been so sure that somebody like Penny was more than capable of treating patients in the right kind of way, with compassion, empathy, and sympathy, but the higher officers made this doubly hard for sincere, well-meaning people to do their jobs adequately.

She couldn't understand how anybody could hope to find the right help for somebody who was so distressed that they didn't feel like there was anything left worth living for any longer.

Melanie had started feeling like this herself, but she found it was a complete eye-opener, and made her realise how dangerous it was to misjudge people in the situation of having found out that they are mentally ill. Maybe some of the staff were bullies, underneath; even the power issue clouded their judgment of the people they were supposed to be helping recover so much more. They needed better listening skills. Rosie's family definitely needed to listen to each other more – if they had only sat down together and really listened to each other in the first place, then maybe they might have been able to avoid the endless trips to A and E.

The family had been dysfunctional for a great deal longer than any of them would have cared to admit. No wonder Melanie had felt pushed to the limits, to the point of suddenly finding she was going beyond her limits. When she had agreed to marry David, she longed for a normal family life more than ever. Her own parents had had their fair share of problems with a turbulent marriage. This was one of her dreams, to have a blissfully happy family life; it was ok to have dreams in life. Having dreams somehow breaks the monotony of the dullness of every day existence. Melanie longed for the stability that she'd lacked throughout her own childhood She vowed that she'd never put her own family through what she'd had to witness through her teens. Just imagine how much more guilty she felt about the effects of her failed relationship with Rosie, not to mention the already mounting deep sense of failure as she started becoming more and more depressed, the more hopeless the situation got.

Every Saturday Melanie had made a futile attempt at trying to arrange a family outing. She ended up having to cope with a crisis situation with Rosie, made doubly difficult because it was next to impossible to get hold of anyone from the hospital team at all at weekends. This made it even harder for Melanie to deal with the already mounting stress problems, as she found herself having to explain the situation time and time again to the duty psychiatrists, once she'd actually managed to get through to a human being on the other end of the line, and not just a recorded message. Instead of taking the family out for a walk by the river on a Saturday afternoon, Saturday afternoons would frequently see them sitting in casualty, with Rosie on the trolley looking forward to nothing except a five-hour wait. It would be doubly frustrating, as most of the medical staff were preoccupied with doing paperwork, leaving their patients in limbo on the trolleys. Why can't the staff have a separate time to concentrate on paperwork, then deal solely with the matter in question, which should be trying to see as many patients as possible, in as short a time as possible. There seems to be a massive loophole in the system somewhere along the line. The patients are being let down by the very people who have the most power to help them. It is so vitally important for every single family with a teenage member to be as open as possible with communication. Rosie had felt so frightened by her psychotic episodes because she didn't believe that she had anyone she could go to talk to, there was absolutely no-one she felt close enough to even begin to understand. She couldn't talk to either of her parents because of all the constant arguing going on in the house. The arguing was making Rosie feel more and more isolated. She'd escape to her bedroom, and then become psychotic, having visions, and hearing her voices. David was the only real escape route – she relied on him to help her maintain what little sanity she had left.

As Melanie realised her daughter had disappeared, she felt she had come to the end of her resources and there was no point in trying to keep the family together any longer. It had gone way beyond all state of repair – once you couldn't trust a person that was it. There could be no relationship there, none whatsoever.

The main issues Melanie was facing was the fact that she had been depressed for a long time – that she'd caused her own problem by becoming too focused on trying to help others deal with their problems. Now, the best thing she could hope for her family would be to let things happen of their own accord. There was simply no other way forward – much as she wanted to keep David, the most loving thing she could do for both Rosie and David would be to let them both go. She had to desert that situation, and be strong enough to be able to let go of them and move forward. There was no alternative. The most crucial thing for Melanie, though, was to put herself first, for a change, and get her strength back. She could do this as a favour to each of them – but she started realising that she put others first all the time, because she was too unhappy inside herself to concentrate on herself, at all.

This was time for real growth, but the single remaining question would be for Melanie herself. Would she be strong enough to move forward, in a bid for freedom and independence? If she had time on her own, she'd be able to find the true person, the true person hidden amidst all the noise and total disruption of a normal existence.

SHOCKING PINK

David couldn't take anything in. Things hadn't been right between him and Melanie for such a long time now, but they had still seemed able to put up a façade of the average middle class 2.4 children scenario, even though the reality couldn't have been anything further than the truth.

All David could think about now was the possibility of losing not just one, but both people he cared about most in the world. He knew how concerned he'd been about Rosie since this latest episode. His main concern had been due to the inadequate care offered to his daughter by the health services that were, in his opinion, woefully inadequate in basic communication skills, not giving enough time to care for the struggling patients. His anger was not misplaced, and it spurred him into action to protect his stepdaughter from herself. He knew she was headed on a slippery downward slope; she had always been her own worst enemy. She was so bound up by whatever was going on around in that confused head of hers that he feared that she wouldn't come out of all this in one piece, this time. She might not even still be alive – he'd seen her when she had had psychotic episodes before, but it was the high episodes which scared her the most, when he'd see her personality changed so completely, that he didn't know who she was any more even though he knew that he was probably the person who was closest to her. He was scared of what she might end up doing, when she became invincible – she'd imagine that she was capable of doing anything, now she'd run off, and it was up to David to rectify the situation he felt responsible for causing. He was, spurred into action by his own feelings of insurmountable guilt. Maybe there might be a way through this time though, by doing his best for Rosie. That was when he decided to make it his mission in life to be her rescuer. But he was trying to rescue his own issues, when he realised that he'd damaged his family beyond repair. Melanie had turned out to be the true rescuer.

David felt a huge amount of righteous anger towards the healthcare professionals, and the healthcare system in general. If the care offered to the family had been adequate in the first place, the family would probably have managed to survive against all the odds, surviving all the battering that fate had thrown at them in the face of mental illness.

They shouldn't have had to spend most of their precious family time coming back to the hospital, only to be completely humiliated by the very staff that were struggling to 'protect' their medical staff from too high a workload. The staff, who should have been attending to their patients instead of sitting at a desk on the ward, doing paperwork, had their priorities, all wrong.

David could quite understand why Rosie had decided to flee from the ward, but he couldn't help feeling a sense of deep anxiety for her safety. She always acted so irrational when she felt she was invincible. This was why she had been sectioned under the Mental Health Act twenty-one times already, and she was still only 14 years old. Every time she was sectioned, it seemed that the police were really no better at knowing how best to handle the situation than the local casualty departments had done on the occasions that he and the family had had to return there, weekend after weekend, full of frustration because of having difficulty getting hold of anyone remotely capable of making coherent sense. No wonder the patients on the wards were acting so oddly. It was completely beyond David how anyone could hope to survive to the next 24 hours as a scientific experiment, all this probing and questioning that they had to go through constantly – digging around past memories in a futile fashion, round and round in circles, going further and further into a completely psychotic mind – how could a stranger have any knowledge of what had happened to another stranger they had only spoken to for twenty minutes? No, in this day and age of enlightenment, there had to be an alternative method of treatment to offer, other than traditional psychiatry, such as creativity, or past life regression David felt sure, from his experiences with intuition regarding other people. Perhaps unresolved unhappiness might have come from a previous existence? Life wasn't black and white; there were too many grey areas, to which even the most highly qualified psychiatrists couldn't possibly have the answer for. The psychosis that he'd seen happen to Rosie on so many occasions…could it be possible that it was a separate life? Sometimes it would seem almost as if the mind had a separate existence all its own. The "psychotic" state of mind was almost as if the mind were coming to life, and having a life all its own.

With all the advancements in medical knowledge David was increasingly distressed and horrified that psychiatry seemed to be at a standstill, and that all the training received by GPs was a general overall picture of a twelve week training period before being let loose in a surgery. Now Rosie had done a runner, it was entirely up to David to make up for the pain and anguish that Rosie had to fight every day of her young life. It had never even occurred to David that Rosie was running away from him, that her feelings of overwhelming guilt because of the 'forbidden' love that she had for him, made her feel so fragile when she was with him, that she had to get away. These questions could only possibly be answered once David had found Rosie, but the events were going to turn around, and bring them back together.

CHARCOAL

Even though Melanie's mind seemed to be nothing but a whirlpool that was twisting and turning, round and round, as her thoughts were spiralling downwards into a mass of confusion, Melanie knew that she needed to turn from the inner confusion, in order to reach the place of some kind of clarity of thought. She needed that clarity because Rosie was in danger, and Melanie's instincts told her that she was the only person who would be able to rescue Rosie from herself and the web of deceit that David had woven around her.

David was slowly starting to become more and more impatient with Rosie, as he realised that she was starting to become more of a liability to him now she was starting to become more psychotic as time went on. "There has to be some way out – some solution." David thought. "I need to be rid of her. I need some way of just getting rid of the burden. It's too much like a millstone around my neck."

David started spicing up his next plan of action in the great master plan.

He'd been doing drugs all the time he'd been on his own with Rosie, but up to now, he'd never actually put Rosie in a situation where she'd been forced to take any, or taken anything without her knowledge. Now, however, it was a different matter. David felt angry. His anger with Rosie began to become extreme. Somehow he had to take revenge on her for all the suffering that the family had had to go through over the years on his stepdaughter's behalf.

Who knows, even his relationship with Melanie could have worked itself out, and taken a turn for the better, had it not been of all the extra pressure on Melanie. All because of Rosie. It was all Rosie's fault. Every single bit of it.

Now David had to make sure that he had his chance to be free from all of it. David hadn't got a conscience. He never felt any remorse about his relationship with Rosie – who knows, maybe if he had then the family might still be together. Although, there again, it might still have proved to be much too late.

At least Rosie tried to help with the cooking – but she was so slow and clumsy. David often felt that she might have well been a severely retarded mentally handicapped person, with a mental age of only four or five years old the way that she behaved, sometimes. Rosie was a hopeless case, because she wasn't able to keep her mind on the job. Frequently, she'd lose track of following even the simplest of recipes, as her voices kept interfering as they tried to distract her. As far as David could see, Rosie was neither use nor ornament. She was a complete burden to everyone around her. David even began to have a sense of total compassion towards his wife, Melanie. He'd never attempted to try to understand the situation from her point of view – ever. But now it seemed, he was picking up the thread of the sense of frustration that Melanie had tried so hard to tell him about so many times – he'd never heard what she was trying to tell him not once, in the last two years of his married life. He'd spent so much of his time avoiding even the remotest opportunity to talk about things openly. That was probably the worst thing that he could have done. He and Melanie had never actually sat down to talk seriously about anything that mattered, not once, over the last four years. Not since David had started the affair with Rosie. Communication had gradually shut down, as David's walls of secrecy had begun to spring up, one by one by one. It seemed the communication that was so desperately needed between them, was springing up more and more with the secret that David had to have, and there were so many secrets, not to mention the biggest secret, the biggest lie of all – which was his relationship with Rosie. That was when the web of deceit was beginning to be spun.

What must it be like, living without a conscience? Maybe the criminal minds never have any conscience in the first place. This drives people to speed up the need for revenge because the real need for remorse becomes the great need. It dampens any sense of guilt or remorse, but more often than not, is there is no conscience; the person is incapable of feeling the remotest sense of remorse, and how can they?

David had felt no pangs of guilt when he'd added the powder to the gravy, as he cooked the Sunday lunch. He felt not one single pang of remorse as he watched Rosie's hallucinations worsen. This time, the hallucinations would prove to be an ally for Rosie. However, David shut himself off from the possibility that the drugs might be causing Rosie's psychotic episodes. But the hallucinations would actually end up doing Rosie a good turn, as it was the voices that would turn the tide and eventually end up turning it in Rosie's favour.

Even the black sheep of the family would have its day. The voices would change the tone of their voice. Instead of the usual, harsh, condemning voice, a new voice sprung up, in the middle of the chaos, into a positive sounding voice, with different qualities of sound, producing a different meaning. That positive voice helped to shed a new light on Rosie's inner perspective. Up to now, she'd almost felt that Melanie was completely against her. Was Rosie's paranoia becoming paranoid?

But even that sensation began fading, as the voices changed, yet again. Sometimes Rosie wondered if there was more than one voice in there. But she was so confused every time she heard even one voice that she couldn't even begin to make any sort of logical conclusion about her thoughts. Perhaps, though, there wasn't really any real reason to be logical. Maybe all that was needed was the time to take a step back and just qualm the fears inside herself. Be more able to listen. How much time does the average person actually spend each day properly withdrawing from the after effects of the outside world, to be able to begin to get in touch with the inner voice? In fact, very rarely. It's a special person who does. In reality, if they can, it's often the mentally ill people who are the ones who are special, more special than a normal person, because they possess special qualities that emerge deeper than anything – deeper qualities than anyone normal would be able to experience. Take David and Melanie, for example, if both of them could have made sure that they had put that kind of activity into their every day lives, then their marriage would have at least had more of a chance of being able to keep dancing along to the same tune of life, instead of dancing to different tunes. There might have been some harmony, instead of disharmony, some unity, instead of disunity. Without Rosie in the picture, David felt strongly that Melanie might have found the happiness that always seemed to be just out of her reach. He hadn't planned to attempt to murder Rosie, just to give her enough drugs to confuse her, with any luck, she just might wander off, get lost, and then flee. David would be able to conclude the working of his master plan.

After lunch that afternoon, Rosie began to feel worse, much worse. She couldn't walk in a straight line, nor could she think straight. Her voices kept getting dimmer and dimmer, Rosie was hopeful that they might fade away in the distance altogether, especially since they weren't even meant to be there, after the E.C.T.

As her inner voices faded, Rosie became aware of a brand-new voice trying to make an appearance. It wasn't a voice that Rosie had ever heard before, either. It actually made her feel as if she were much, much stronger, not weaker; Rosie also had a flash of inspiration. She'd never looked at the situation from Melanie's point of view. She'd been too ill to even think about somebody else, let alone understand whatever might be happening. The one thing Rosie had been aware of was that Melanie had always been the one who had been there, trying to pick up the pieces for Rosie. She'd never been aware that Melanie might have had to make great personal sacrifices in order to be able to do things. Rosie had spent most of her life fighting against Melanie. Now she began to realise that Melanie had actually been on her side all along. Had Rosie lost all her chances of being able to redeem her relationship with Melanie? As the situation between her and David got more and more tense, she found herself longing for Melanie's calming influence. She was so scared that she'd driven it away. Perhaps there would never be another chance to make her peace. Rosie couldn't understand why David was keeping his distance from her. She needed support from someone. Her hallucinations were really troubling her. Suddenly she had the thought that she could be the one in control over David, AND her voices. The voices kept returning with just one, single, returning thought: "KILL".

As David was starting to do the washing-up that Sunday afternoon, Rosie had already gone into the kitchen to find a carving knife. She stood behind David who was totally unaware of her presence, with the knife raised. David discovered it before Rosie had the chance to bring the knife plunging down. He grabbed her, bundled her off into the bedroom, locking the door. He knew his stepdaughter's auditory hallucinations had finally got the victory. But he was not about to give Rosie the freedom she deserved, and that was rightfully hers.

Melanie had had to fight the authorities at the hospital to try to get help to find Rosie and David. She felt as if she were banging her head against a brick wall. It was up to Melanie to locate where the missing runaways were. The only hope was that Rosie might have access to David's mobile phone, but given the circumstances, with the way that Rosie felt about using a mobile phone when she was ill, this would be extremely unlikely. Something David had mentioned about wanting to go to Amsterdam to paint kept coming back into Melanie's thoughts as she mulled over where the missing pair might be. She was unable to convince the authorities to pay for her to bring Rosie home. They refused to listen to Melanie's pleas for help, refusing to accept responsibility for the disappearance and insisting that Melanie provide her own finances to search for her missing relatives – they washed their hands of the situation.

Melanie felt trapped. She'd somehow have to borrow the money from somewhere. She ended up approaching her father for help, after much arguing, he reluctantly agreed to lend her the money on the understanding that she would pay it back as soon as she could. Melanie hated having to be in the position of borrowing money from any one. But she knew Rosie needed her.

Fortunately, The Police had been more than willing to be helpful in this case, and had agreed to come abroad with Melanie, once they had made contact with Rosie, especially as they were keen to question Rosie about what had happened with Jamie McBride.

David had finally agreed to let Rosie out of the bedroom, but not before piling her high with drinks spiced with Cannabis. He made sure every single door and window in the house was locked. He watched, sombrely, as she grew weaker and weaker, until she decided to go to bed, as she didn't feel well. He took advantage of her weakness, and used it to get her to sleep with him. She said "yes", but David knew that it wasn't really Rosie saying this. She was under the influence of both drink and drugs.

Rosie was barely conscious, and completely unaware that David was on top of her making love to her. There was a loud knock on the door, making David jump. He opened the door to Melanie and two policemen who abruptly handcuffed him and forced him to show them where Rosie was. They carried an unconscious Rosie into the police car to escort her to the hospital to recover, before making the journey back to Great Britain with Melanie, but without David.

David had been left out in the cold for good.

Claire De Lune.

David found himself spending longer hours staying behind after class to paint, as he was much too lonely in the staff flat that he was staying in on campus. It was much easier for him to work in the studio than to have to spend hours having to face the prospect of working alone. He had a creative outlet, and could switch off from his recurring thoughts while he was choosing his colours. He found it most beneficial to concentrate on just one colour at a time – that seemed to help him to achieve a fresh, clarifying thought. He wanted to be in the countryside, not in the town, but as there was no prospect of getting to the country, he had to content himself with painting the images of the wild flowers that grew up the grassy banks in his mind's eye. David loved the dancing poppies scattered around in the golden hay. He could almost feel the fresh, summer breeze blowing through their delicate petals. As he stood by his easel, stains of one of his favourite piano pieces, by Debussy "The Girl With The Flaxen Hair" suddenly drifted from one of the practise rooms. He pricked up his ears, relaxing totally as he moved his brush up and down the canvas, following the rhythms and tonal qualities of the silk sounds coming from the phrases of the beautiful music.

David was totally captivated by the tonal quality of the sounds.

The feeling of deja-vu was beginning to become more and more evident, as David and Claire spent more time together. They had taken to meeting up with each other every evening after David had finished his painting. To begin with, they just went for a quiet drink together, David sensed that Claire was isolated and lonely, and wanted to help her find her way through her isolation, by offering her an outlet for some kind of social life. However, this was now starting to become more sinister, and he found himself taking advantage of the fact that she was lonely and isolated, manipulating it in order to gratify his own needs.

As is often the case with people who seem unable to have any kind of a conscience, David was one of those people who didn't even notice, or care when he was starting to take advantage of somebody else. Claire's attraction to David had started becoming a full-scale infatuation, somehow, she found herself getting caught up in the excitement by the fact that David appeared to be falling head over heels in love with her. Actually, no – it wasn't really falling in love, it was more like an experience of love at first sight, or so it would seem. Claire had no idea that this man, who seemed so transfixed by her, was incapable of caring about anyone else except himself. She was in for a rude awakening. The awakening happened gradually, as they started spending time together in David's flat. The secrets were beginning to be let out of Pandora's Box.

David sent Claire a text message on her mobile while he was painting. He had to finish his work first, before arranging to meet her in the pub. So he innocently suggested that she meet up with some of the other music students who would already be in there before he got there. As Claire read his text message, she was in a quandary about what to do. She hated going into crowded places on her own. The thought was absolutely terrifying for her. It had taken all her courage to arrange to meet David, let alone meet a load of people she didn't know in a crowded bar on her own. She struggled with her insecurities as she tried to work out the best plan of action. Wouldn't it be better to give tonight a miss? Then she knew she couldn't handle the possibility of not being able to see David for another 24 hours at least. The longing to spend as much time as possible together got the better of her. She knew she had to break out of her shell eventually. This time it had to be now, or never. So she sent David a message that she would go to the bar and wait there for him for half an hour but no longer.

Claire could hear her heart thumping loudly as she pushed the door open. She could see crowds of people standing near the bar. She panicked at the thought of having to fight her way through them to ask for a drink on her own. As she looked around the crowded bar, assessing the situation, her biggest impulse was to turn on her heels and run. But there was something that kept her there, no matter how much she wanted to take flight. There was an open-mic performance happening she could hear somebody playing the keyboards, which made her curious. Curiosity killed the cat; she decided to try to get a closer look at whoever was playing. They weren't at all bad. She realised, as she got closer, that it was one of the fellow – music students from her year. Well maybe in that case, there might be a few of the others around, it was so busy in there it would be easy to miss a large group of people, huddled together with their backs to you. Her eyes scanned the tables hoping to see some familiar faces. She was in luck. One of the girls in her ear-training group waved to her and beckoned her over, pointing to the seat next to her. Claire felt tremendously relieved when she sat down next to Sabrina.   "This is an unexpected pleasure," said Sabrina. "What brings you here tonight, then? Have you decided to have a break for a change? I thought you were much too busy to have a social life."

"I'm meeting someone in here a bit later" said Claire.

"Who's the lucky fella then?" asked Sabrina,

"What makes you think I'm meeting a male friend? I haven't got time for developing friendships, I'm way too busy."

"That is usually the reason for girls to turn up in a bar on their own" Sabrina told her, "You don't usually come anywhere near any of us. But hey, it's good to see you. Sit down here with us, and we'll buy you a drink, won't we?" she nudged one of the male students sitting next to her.

"Yes, yes. Of course, what are you having?" he asked Claire.

"Just orange juice, please. Thank you, that's kind." She sat down next to Sabrina. "Are you sure we can't tempt you into having something a bit stronger?" he asked.

"No- that'll be just fine." Claire waited until he had gone to the bar before asking "Who's he?"

"That's Martin, he's a fantastic pianist too. God, he's so lucky, He's got such big hands, and he can play anything and everything that I can't manage. People with big hands are so lucky, they have it made. How do you manage, you are quite small really, aren't you?"

"Actually I don't find it matters too much." said Claire, "I seem able to find a way of playing most things. I sometimes wish that I had been a man, though, because of their strength when it comes to playing. I wish I could play Beethoven in such a powerful way. Anyway, you haven't introduced me to the others yet; I'd like to meet them properly."

"Oh, excuse me," said Sabrina. "Well, these are some of the art students, who are working on the art and music project that we are doing at the moment. This is John, Paul, and Richard."

"I'm meeting one of the art tutors in here, actually." Claire told them. Richard and John looked at each other.

"Are you sure you know what you are doing? It's not a great idea to spend time alone with somebody who has got such a bad reputation, you know."

"I am not sure I know what you mean." Claire found that she was starting to feel more awkward,

"Well, it won't be that long before you'll find out – trust us" Richard said. "Ah, here he comes."

David had walked into the bar, and was standing in the room, obviously looking for somebody. His face lit up like a Christmas tree when he saw Claire.

"So THAT'S who you're spending time with, then" said Sabrina. "Are you sure that you know what you are doing?"

"Should I be, he seems to be a lovely man," Claire told her, not really understanding why Richard and John had started choking on their beers. "Have I said something wrong?" Claire asked, awkwardly.

"No – no, not at all, just be careful, you'll need to watch yourself, though" said Richard.

"I don't like your insinuations." Claire was feeling rather upset by now and indicated to David to find them somewhere to sit alone, away from the group. She stood up to go over to meet David, but the room suddenly started going around in circles as her head swam. David noticed, and came over to her straight away. "Are you ok?" David asked.

"I'm fine, just fine, let's go." Claire told him, so David guided her to a quiet corner over on the other side of the bar, but not before Claire had noticed the others were sniggering.

"Is anything wrong?" she asked him.

"Not at all, they are just a bunch of immature idiots," said David, "I wanted to ask you to come around to my flat this evening, would you like to?"

"That is really sweet of you" Claire told him "Of course I would like to. Shall we go there now?" She started shaking as she stood up, and had to sit down again.

"What's wrong, don't you feel well?" David asked her.

"As it happens, I do feel rather strange" said Claire. "I will probably feel much better for a rest "

"Come on, let's go home." David guided her out of the bar, but she was still feeling sick and giddy. "I tell you what, I have a coffee-maker back home, I'll make you a strong black coffee. That will help."

David's flat was on the top floor of an old Victorian house in a leafy suburb in Camberwell Green. The house was extremely atmospheric; as soon as one entered it you felt that you were entering into a different time. David had tried to recapture the Victorian atmosphere with the way that he had furnished the flat. He'd decorated it in cream, and bought maroon velvet curtains, as well as having a comfortable pine rocking chair by the open fire. He showed Claire the cream sofa, and told her to go and sit down while he went into the kitchen to make some coffee.

Claire was fascinated by all the beautiful paintings on the wall, which she realised, were David's own work. She couldn't believe how talented he was as she looked at the different scenes from nature, which represented the different seasons, Spring, Summer, Autumn and Winter. After a while, David returned to join her on the sofa. She soon found that she was more interested in him than in the coffee.

As they sat closely together, it was harder and harder for Claire to resist the temptation. She found herself wanting to become closer and closer to this man. She still felt shy and exposed as she picked up on the warmth from the physical closeness, as it seemed he was drawing her closer to him. They were sitting so closely together, their knees were touching. David decided to take a chance, and suddenly bent his head and kissed her warm, sweet lips, rendering her completely helpless. Suddenly the kissing became frantic, as they touched each other's tongues. David stroked her thighs rubbing her skirt against them. She felt his body through the crisp white shirt. He picked her up, and carried her to the floor, where he lay on top of her, stroking her hair, sending her into ecstasy. They started to roll round and round on the floor, kissing and kissing and kissing. David could feel himself becoming so aroused that he feared for the consequences. Claire was rubbing his penis with her hands, starting to make it go harder, and he just couldn't cope, the chemistry was so overwhelming. He'd never made love to somebody that he was so completely in love with before in his entire life. He suddenly knew it had to stop here, because it would spoil the magic that was already there between them. "Darling…" he whispered in her ear, "It's too soon. Don't you think we're going too fast?"

"I want you."

"Yes, my love, I want you too … but this thing between us, I can't handle it. I'm scared."

"But I HAVE to have you." Claire told him. That was enough for David. He started to remove Claire's clothes, not slowly, but ripping them off like a savage animal. They caressed every part of each other; David could feel Claire's silk skin melting into his. He started getting warmer and warmer and warmer, moving on top of Claire faster and faster. Claire grabbed him, rolling over, so that she was the one on top, kissing and kissing until David had to break away, unable to breathe for the excitement. He was conscious that this moment would be over in a flash, lost forever. It did come to a close, but he stroked Claire's beautiful blonde hair as they lay in each other's arms, cuddling each other, savouring every single, precious moment.

"I wish it could stay like this forever" Claire whispered, "I wish I never had to go".

"You don't" David said, "Why don't you stay? There's nothing to stop you."

"I don't know whether it's such a good idea to rush things." Claire said. "I don't really know you that well."

"All the more reason to spend as much time as we can getting to know all about each other then, my darling." said David. "I don't think I can hold out long enough until I see you again if you went home now. Please stay with me." He begged, making Claire's heart melt.

"All right then, I will – so long as I manage to keep to my normal routine ok."

They curled up in each other's arms, cuddling each other until they both fell asleep.

Claire woke up the next morning, panicking. It took her quite some time to work out where she was. As she started waking up, her instincts told her that she wasn't at home. She realised she was sleeping on her own, when she saw that David's half of the bed was empty.

David had woken up earlier than Claire, and had already been out of the house. He always went out early in the morning to visit one of his drug-dealing friends to make sure that his daily supply was big enough. It was best to go to find them first thing in the morning, because there was hardly anybody around then, who could cause trouble for them. He' d always come back to the flat, and prepare the heroin to put into the needle, in order to inject himself with enough to keep him going for the rest of the day. This was the only time of day that he would be guaranteed peace and quiet. He usually went to the toilet, locked the door, and injected himself privately; it was the only place he knew no one would find out about what he'd done, because he could flush the evidence away. This morning, though, he'd forgotten to lock the door.

Claire went to the toilet as quickly as possible. She knew she would have to search for David immediately after she'd finished getting dressed. The toilet door was still slightly ajar, so she pushed it open. As she pushed it open, her mouth just fell open in absolute horror. David was there, sticking a needle into his arm. Claire shut the door quickly behind her, fearful of discovery, but had decided not to let on to David that she'd seen what he was up to. She made a conscious decision not even to drop a hint to him that there was anything wrong. But she couldn't hide how upset she felt. She was distraught. The person she loved was causing himself serious damage, but it was even worse than that, he was KILLING himself, willingly.
She tried to keep quiet, but she loved David too much to allow anything to hurt him.
She knew then, that this was love, because she knew that she would do everything in her power to stop anything, or anyone from hurting this man, who she now knew was the love of her life. She would live, breath, and DIE for him. Claire didn't really know what her best course of action was. She knew she should tell David that she was well aware of what was going on, but she didn't feel secure enough in her new relationship to risk losing David. She just knew that she couldn't bear losing him.

With the way things were looking, especially with what she'd just discovered about him, there was a very strong chance that she might end up losing him forever, as it was. He hadn't seen her standing there, so she decided to keep her mouth shut for now, at least. She could bide her time with this one.

Unfortunately, though, she might have found herself able to save her own life, had she spoken out sooner. She had no idea about the implications of the twist of fate that not speaking about this would prove to have on her entire life. But what had happened that morning had started a cycle of hatred towards anything to do with drugs. She couldn't bear to see the man she loved so deeply injecting himself, daily – at this stage she hadn't realised that this is what she 'd be contending with every day she and David spent together, the price to pay for the sheer bliss and happiness they had together was far to high, and wasn't even worth the fatal consequences.

Nocturne

Melanie and Rosie had managed to maintain some kind of normality when they had finally arrived home. Life went on much the same a usual, except that, on the whole, there was more closeness between Rosie and Melanie than there had ever been. Having the secret out in the open meant that they could begin to get to know one another all over again, without becoming entangled by the web of deceit getting in the way. Rosie had been manipulated by someone else's selfishness all along, which didn't help the barriers come down, that should never have been there in the first place.

But the newfound honesty between Melanie and Rosie was almost too good to be true. There had to be a spanner in the works. Rosie started to settle down, as she felt safer as time went on, and she managed to get back to some kind of normality and routine, without feeling that she had something to hide from other people, all the time. It was too perfect to last. Rosie realised that she would need to keep an eye on her menstrual cycle after she had come home. This was a particularly worrying time for her, as it meant that she was overly anxious, waiting for the time of the month to appear, with baited breath. It was now nearly three months since Rosie had been brought back home, and there were still no signs of her monthly periods happening at their usual time. Rosie had always had a vague feeling of panic at the possibility that she might end up becoming pregnant as a result of her relationship with David. But because she was so young, she knew that there was no way that she could talk openly to anyone at all about her under-age sexual relationship with her step-dad. She was petrified she'd get both of them, and especially David, into serious trouble once the whole truth was out there. But as the third month of missing her period was rapidly approaching, she knew she had to have help, and fast. How could she possibly be in a position to have a baby at her age? These were exceptional circumstances that she was facing, because the father of her baby was a family member, although not a blood relative, this meant that this would have far greater an impact on the rest of their lives. After what they had all just come through, she couldn't put Melanie through any more torture. She was still fearful that Melanie was slowly becoming more and more unstable as time went on, surely it would only take one more thing to push her too far over the edge? Rosie didn't want to be the one to be responsible for causing somebody else to have a nervous breakdown.

Rosie found herself in a quandary. She didn't know where to turn for help and support. The situation she'd got herself into meant that she was much more vulnerable than most. It was an impossibly enough situation for anyone who found themselves becoming pregnant when they were so terribly young, but it was just too much to have to face the prospect of carrying your step-father's child inside you for nine months, with far reaching consequences on your relationship with your mother, who would usually have been your main support system under the normal circumstances. Rosie was well aware that her family had lost its sense of normality a long time ago – long before all this happened. Now she couldn't even approach her mother for the sort of experienced counselling that she should have been able to have straight forward access to in such a situation. Maybe the most important thing she had to do next was to go to see the doctor. But she wished that she didn't have to go to see the family's GP – she was fearful of discovery. There had to be another way to make sure that her business stayed her own private business. It wasn't anything to do with anyone else in the world. She wanted it to be David's business. But it was too much to expect that wishes to even come true.

Rosie was starting to feel like she was walking around carrying the weight of the whole world on her young shoulders. But time was now starting to run out, and she was becoming more and more conscious of this. It was time for action. All the contemplating in the world she could possibly have done alone, had been done. Taking a deep breath, she picked up the phone and booked an appointment to see the GP later that week. Three days to wait. It wasn't really that long now, in retrospect.

On the day of the appointment, Rosie lied to Melanie about where she was going. This was something else that Rosie hated doing. She found herself constantly having to cover up for herself because she was trapped into doing things that made her feel uncomfortable. Because of having no one to ask advice from, she felt that she had no choice except lying her way out of trouble. David had taught her that was the best way to get by in life, but as she faced this new situation, she knew all her hopes and dreams would be blown to the winds.

On the morning of the appointment, Rosie felt she wanted the floor of the surgery's waiting room to open up and swallow her whole. She had never felt so uncomfortable in her life, wondering whether any of her family's neighbours might have booked an appointment to see their GP on the same morning. So far, so good – thankfully there were very few people waiting to see the doctor first thing in the morning, Rosie was thankful for small mercies. She had never been so relieved in her life when the doctor opened the door and called her name. Rosie had done her best to make sure that she'd see a doctor who wasn't the one who was attending to every other member of her family.

Nervously, Rosie walked into the doctor's room. Out of the corner of her eye, she could see children's toys in the corner. Her heart missed a beat, for just a split second as she realised what she was about to ask the doctor to do for her. She suddenly saw a picture in her mind's eye of two young toddlers, a boy and a girl, playing quietly in the corner. The image was imprinted on her brain. She felt that she must be the most evil person on the earth, having to ask the doctor the questions she now had no choice but to ask. She had to ask – for sanity's sake.

"What seems to be the problem?" asked Dr Green.

Dr Green was tall and slim, with dark hair, in her early thirties. Rosie noticed that she was married. She couldn't be very old. Rosie wondered if she had children of her own.

"I've missed my period two months in a row, and I did one of those home pregnancy tests, you know the sort I mean – the ones where the strip turns blue if you are pregnant."

"What happened?"

"It was blue and I'm certain I'm pregnant. My body feels different. I know I'm changing, that there's something else growing inside me."

"How old are you?" came the question of all questions. Rosie felt tempted to take the usual, easy way out and lie to the doctor about her age. It would be easy enough. So many people always said they thought she was at least sixteen. But now wasn't the time for lies. Whatever the cost, the truth must be told.

"I'm fourteen" Dr Green looked shocked.

"How many weeks pregnant do you think you are? What do you want to do?"

"I'm sure I'm not three months yet," Rosie faltered.

"Have you told your parents, we can't really do very much else for you, we prefer to be able to talk to them as well as you, if possible"

"No, and I don't want them to know anything about this," Rosie said, "They are going through a very difficult time. It wouldn't be fair"

"What do you want to happen?" asked the doctor.

"I want things to be back to normal, I just don't feel normal. I have never felt normal since I had that wretched E.C.T. I can't remember things; I don't feel like a normal human being. I can't possibly have a baby now. Please can you arrange for me to have an abortion as soon as possible," she pleaded.

"I'm sorry, but I am not able to discuss the matter with you any further. I can't deal with your case, I can't advise you, it's against my principals, you will have to find another doctor, and you need two doctor's signatures before anyone will be able to agree to perform a termination, it would have been much more of a help if you had come to see me sooner. Time isn't on our side, anymore, I will have to pass you on to someone else. I'm not willing to take your case on."

"But how much time have we got?" wailed Rosie, "It takes so long to get an appointment, what happens if I am more than twelve weeks pregnant?"

"I can book you in as an emergency case with one of my colleague's tomorrow." Dr Green told her. "You'll have to book the appointment at reception on your way out".

It was clear that she hadn't realised how much mental distress she had caused Rosie by putting her under so much more stress. Rosie's anxiety levels were now soaring sky high out of all proportion. She was shaking like a leaf as she stood by the desk at reception.

"I have to book an appointment with another doctor for tomorrow, please"

"Dr Green has already rung through to inform us about this situation, there's only one appointment tomorrow, with Dr Radcliffe, and he's your normal family GP, isn't he? Do you mind about that?" Rosie had started becoming hotter and hotter, feeling very sick and faint, her knees had started shaking. She fainted in front of the receptionist, and the long queue of patients who were waiting their turn to book appointments.

She was aware of being surrounded by a sea of faces. The surgery nurse was bending over her, giving her a glass of water. "Is there anyone we can call for you, what about your mother?" she asked Rosie.

"No, no, no, thanks, I'm fine. I'll be fine; really, I just want to get home."

"Do you want us to call you a cab?"

"I haven't any money." Rosie told them, "Anyway, it's best for me if I have a walk in the fresh air. I'm sure that will help" As she stood up Rosie started to feel sick. She released she was going to have another bout of the morning sickness which had started happening more often. "I'm going to be sick" she informed the nurse, who helped her to the ladies toilets. Rosie looked pale when she came.

After Rosie washed her face and had had a drink of the fresh, cold water, she started to walk. It wasn't really such a very long walk, but this morning felt like the longest walk she had ever been on.

She had never felt so alone in the whole of her young life.

Dr Green felt upset for the rest of the morning, after she had refused to help Rosie, but in spite of this, she knew that there was no way that she could feel comfortable about giving advice to someone over such a delicate matter, that she felt unable to deal with on personal, moral grounds. Dr Green had had her own agenda when it came to the issue of abortion.

She and her husband had had enormous difficulty conceiving a child due to her husband's low sperm count. They'd have to decide whether to apply to be able to adopt a baby or to go for IVS treatment – both of them wanted a family. They had spent a great deal of money trying treatment after treatment, which always ended up becoming a major disappointment. Dr Green was a healthy young woman, and they had eventually become successful, she'd been over the moon to discover that she was finally pregnant.

The precariousness of the situation had made her value the important things in life more carefully. She found that having to deal with those of her women patients, who wanted to have an abortion, subsequently was one of the most distressing aspects of her very demanding job. Dr Green knew that it was best not to become emotionally entangled with individual cases, but this issue meant it was impossible for her not to feel angry when some people evidently showed that they were simply not ready for the responsibility of having a child, by the very fact that they had turned up asking for an abortion in the first place. Dr Green had made a conscious decision, that she would automatically pass on a patient to one of her colleagues – it would be the same for everyone. So it wasn't anything personal against Rosie, but she was concerned about Rosie's emotional well being, especially since Rosie had spoken to her about how fragile she had been feeling since she had had the E.C.T.

Dr Green was feeling so upset herself, but she needed to discuss the moral ethics involved with one of her colleagues. She saw nothing wrong in discussing the general topic of how to handle needy patients. It didn't have to become a situation of breaking patient confidentiality. So later that morning, she decided to meet Dr Radcliffe for a quiet drink, and a working lunch. Dr Radcliffe was probably the best person that could help Rosie. He knew the family's psychiatric history much better than any of his other colleagues. But he was a specialist in dealing with psychiatry, and very much more aware of the implications of such a situation on a person who had the kind of problems that Rosie's family were coping with.

"I am so glad to be able to talk to somebody," Dr Green told him.

"Don't worry, Valerie, It's best to get these things off your chest. People forget that we doctors are only human beings too – we can only cope with so much. You sound like you have had quite a morning, why are you so worried?"

"This happens to be one of the most difficult parts of my job." Dr Green told him.

"I try not to become emotionally involved with my patients, but this morning was different. This particular situation is especially delicate. I tried to get the patient to talk to her parents, but she refused. I can't say too much for fear of breaking patient confidentiality. But every time anyone asks for an abortion, I feel like the most evil person on earth, that I'm playing God. When one of the patients has gone through with a termination, which, by the way, is ALWAYS against my better judgment, it's the after-effects of the operation, the emotional distress, and the guilt that I have to deal with when the patient comes back to see me after the event."

"I can understand your concerns for this particular case," said Dr Radcliffe. "But our priority is to be accessible to our patients, never mind our own issues. What would happen if somebody felt you were the only person they felt they would be able to relate to? Would that still stand?"

"I see what you mean. It's important to deal with this kind of issue from an objective angle. The best we can do for someone is to give them the right guidance in making the right choice for them, but it is so difficult to be impartial" Dr Green told him.

"I think our biggest problem is that if a patient comes with a particular request, and are told 'no, we can't help' then they will feel that we don't take them seriously, and then the danger will be that they won't talk to anybody else. I realise how difficult it is for somebody with mental health difficulties anyway – it's so easy to be judgmental and think there is no way that they should have got into that situation in the first place, okay, it's an indication that they are not ready for that kind of responsibility at all…but then one could argue that we are being prejudiced against them, assuming that they are not intelligent. No wonder people feel as if they are being patronised. Have I done the right thing?" said Dr. Green

"Yes. I think so. Let me sort it out tomorrow. Will you be able to sign a form at least, if the person is under age, they'll need two doctors to sign the form before they can go ahead with anything"

"No, I'm sorry. That's something that I just can't agree to. What about one of the other doctors in the practice?"

"Leave it to me. You look like you need a break." Said Dr Radcliffe. "We'll sort things out tomorrow."

Indigo

When Rosie woke the next morning, she felt that she couldn't possibly feel more miserable than she already did, but now she was engulfed by a feeling of complete dread on top of it. She had reached the stage of realising that she was the only one who could do something about the way that she responded to whatever knocks life chose to throw at her. It was her decision whether she spent her life feeling miserable, or not. Spending life totally miserable has to be a waste, when you can choose to be happy, anyway, come what may.

Maybe it would help matters if she approached this situation differently. Perhaps there had to be a way round this that she could approach positively instead of negatively. But this would involve a conscious effort on her part to free herself from the negative thought patterns that she'd spent the best part of the last few years battling against Well, this was a war that she was going to win. She knew she could have the victory that was only just out of reach. One day, if she could only resolve this dilemma then there would be no reason on earth why she couldn't make the most of the rest of her life. She was only fourteen years old, after all.

Fourteen, only fourteen and expecting a baby. Suddenly this seemed to be a bigger problem than climbing Mount Everest. But the answer lay in the hands of the doctor who she'd be talking to in less than thirty minutes from now. She hoped and prayed that Dr Radcliffe would be in a good mood this morning. Rosie needn't have worried. Fortunately for her, Dr Radcliffe had already decided that he was going to be bright and cheerful with all his patients. He firmly believed that if the doctors were happy and positive, as well as being approachable, if they succeeded in sending at least one of their patients away happy, then they would have succeeded in doing a good day's work.

"Come in" he said, as Rosie knocked on the door, gingerly. "Do sit down, and make yourself comfortable, my dear" He said, kindly. "There's no need for me to ask you what the matter is, but there are a few points that I'd like to be certain that you really understand properly, before we can go ahead and make any more arrangements. Hopefully, there'll be absolutely nothing at all to worry about, you just need two signatures, and an appointment with the pregnancy advisory service, which will book you an appointment, but hopefully that will only be a last resort. Now, I am surprised you haven't brought your mother with you. We really prefer to be able to speak to the parents of a young person who is under age"

"My mother doesn't know I'm here," Rosie told him. "She doesn't know I'm pregnant. She's had a lot to cope with lately, actually doctor, I'm really worried that she might end up having to go into a mental hospital herself; she's been so down just recently. I don't want to make everything worse for her than is absolutely necessary, and I don't want to be the person that causes her to have a nervous breakdown"

Dr Radcliffe looked surprised. "Is your mother that bad?"
"Yes, but I'm sure she'll be back to normal soon." Rosie told him "At least, I hope so"
"So, how are you as far as hearing your voices is concerned at the moment? Let's see – you had the E.C.T. recently, didn't you? Hopefully things have improved in that direction, since then?"

"Well, this is what I can't understand. I thought that I wouldn't hear the voices ever again, after the troatment, but that's not really been the case, and they still trouble me from time to time. The thing that really worries me is that I feel I may be going mad – because I just don't seem able to remember very large chunks of my past – like memories from my childhood which used to be really important to me, for instance. I was hoping I might be starting to remember more than I have been able to, by now."

"It depends on the individual patient actually. Some people find they lose their memory for longer periods of time than others. It also depends whether they have anything that they subconsciously choose not to be able to remember at all – but of course they are not aware that's what is happening to them. I think you'd feel happier if you speak to your parents, surely?"

"No, there's a very good reason for that. I'd still rather they didn't know. You won't say anything to them, will you?"

"That depends on whether we feel you are capable of making a responsible decision, with all the facts in front of you, and that our decision isn't affected by your condition in any way. We also need to be certain that you might want to choose the option of having your baby adopted. There are so many couples out there who are desperate to have a baby of their own, who can't."

"I've already made up my mind about that, before I came," said Rosie "I could never go through being pregnant for nine months and then end up having to sign my baby over to complete strangers."

"So why is there such a problem with speaking to your parents?"

"I already told you – my mother is unstable at the moment, I think she might become ill herself if she finds herself having to contend with any more shocks. This could very well end up destroying our entire family."

"One of my other colleagues will sign the paper for you, in that case, Rosie. I know you are an intelligent young woman. It's helpful to me that I have known you and the family for such a long time because it has helped me to see that people with mental health difficulties are often very gifted, intelligent people, who are probably more sensitive than most people are. Which is why I have decided that you are perfectly capable of making a clear-headed, responsible decision about this, it seems to me that you are actually making the most responsible choice that's open to you at the moment, because I can tell that you have given the far-reaching consequences for everyone concerned, a lot of thought. Let me go and get my colleague to sign this, and I will sign it too, then we'll sort out an appointment with the pregnancy advisory service, who are more used to dealing with young girls of your age in your position than I am able to."

"Thank you so much for understanding." Rosie breathed a sigh of relief. Now, perhaps, she might stand some chance of her life getting back to normal.

"I wouldn't be a good doctor if I didn't listen to my patients properly, and treat them as individuals" Dr Radcliffe told her. "It's all very well having all the medical qualifications in the world, if you don't treat your patients like human beings, and not a number on the computer system."

"I couldn't agree more" Said Rosie, wholeheartedly.

"Good luck Rosie. I'm sure everything will turn out all right in the end," said the kindly doctor.

"I certainly hope so. Oh gosh, I certainly hope so," Rosie thought to herself, as she walked down the road, feeling considerably less worried than she had when she'd arrived at the doctor's surgery earlier that morning.

Rosie went for her appointment at the pregnancy advice centre later on that week. She found herself sitting opposite a kindly lady, who seemed to be more than willing to spend time listening to her, and seemed experienced enough to understand that she needed reassurance from somebody to quell her fears.

"How can you be sure you're pregnant?" was the first question that she was asked.

"I did the test at home."

"So you think it was a reliable result, then?"

"I haven't had a period for the last two months, and I have started feeling sick every morning," said Rosie.

"Are you having any cravings for strange combinations of food?" asked the pregnancy advisor.

"No, but I can't drink tea and coffee without throwing up any more." Rosie told her.

"What do you want from this situation then, what about the father, does he know, and will he be able to offer you some support?" this question suddenly made Rosie see how hopeless the situation was.

"Did you realise that I am only fourteen years old?" she asked the advisor.

"I wouldn't have guessed… you look much older. I would have said that you were at least 16."

"That causes me most of my problem with the opposite sex." Rosie told her. "They never seem to hear when I tell them I am under age. By the time things got to that point, it's one way too far beyond the boundaries for anyone to stop. There's something else. The person who is the father of my baby must never know. He absolutely MUSTN'T find out. There are too many people's lives at risk".

"Had it ever occurred to you that he might want to know…? To have the opportunity to support you and his child, fairly and squarely? He might be able to support you financially at the very least".

"I wish it was that easy," said Rosie. "But it just isn't, and I just can't tell you why – I can't. There's another reason for wanting to arrange a termination. I have a mental illness; I hear voices all the time. I don't know if it can be passed on to my baby, but it's hell to live with and I wouldn't wish the condition on my worst enemy." The counsellor was one of those caring people. Rosie had been very lucky in finding helpful healthcare professionals.

"I understand, but having a termination isn't something that we feel happy about recommending anyone to have, unless there is simply no other solution. Would you consider having the baby adopted? It would be able to go to a childless couple in a stable relationship. They'd be able to offer your baby a good home and a stable future" Rosie knew this would be impossible. She knew that she had strong maternal instincts, the same as any other woman, and there was no way that she would be able to go all the way through nine months of a pregnancy, go through all the pain of a thirteen hour long labour, and finally actually see and hold the baby knowing that all she'd end up with would be holding nothing in her empty arms. She knew now that this was something she'd never forgive herself for, for the rest of her life. She also knew that David wasn't likely to want to be involved in their child's upbringing. She knew that he'd be a totally irresponsible father; she'd probably end up a homeless single mother, wandering the streets with her unwanted baby, feeling unprotected and unloved. The consequences were too dire. She couldn't do it. It was easier to end the pregnancy than to go through all that. If she had a baby she'd want to be a proper mother, have a nice house, and a loving husband, to complete the package. Now wasn't the time to start a family. It just wasn't right, not at fourteen.

"I have thought this through, and keep thinking it through, until I end up feeling like I am going mad with indecision." Rosie told her. "I'm insisting now, NOT asking, that you book me for an abortion as soon as possible. There's still time left. It's not twelve weeks yet, surely?"
"I hope you won't regret this decision for the rest of your life" said the counsellor, shaking her head, sadly. "You should see some of the girls after they have had the operation. We are always picking up the pieces. They end up totally traumatised. Can't I speak to your mother, at least?" Rosie looked startled.
"NO, no, no…Please don't, you mustn't…She must not ever find out, I swear she mustn't".

The anxiety of carrying this burden that a fourteen year old was much too immature to cope with suddenly became more apparent. The counsellor started realising just how young Rosie was; she wished there was another way. But every time the counsellor had to pass the forms to agree to arrange a termination for a young person, she'd beat herself up about it. Sometimes she couldn't cope with the stress of her job. Reluctantly, she handed Rosie the form. The second form she'd signed in the last six months that would end up with far-reaching consequences. Rosie couldn't help feeling just the tiniest pang of regret as she walked out of the door with an appointment made for the termination.

The fateful day was now a definite black mark by the date in her diary. 22nd APRIL had a black spot marked against it, in her diary. It was only ten days to wait, but it felt more like waiting for ten years. Having to keep absolutely quiet about what was going to happen to her within the next week, as the days went on, was becoming unbearable for Rosie to cope with. She was finding it hard enough to keep her pregnancy hidden from view as it was, she always had to be sure to get up earlier than Melanie, because of the morning sickness that was now starting to happen every day. She'd spend at least twenty minutes throwing up in the bathroom. Melanie had begun to worry that Rosie was starting to suffer from some of the side effects from her psychiatric medication. Sometimes the drugs would cause nausea. Fortunately for Rosie, it didn't occur to Melanie that she had become pregnant.

Rosie had had to spend a considerable amount of time planning out exactly what she was going to tell Melanie the day that she had to go into hospital to have her operation. She'd made up a story about being invited to a friend's house to stay the night. As it was her friend's birthday Melanie did become a little suspicious that there was something not quite right about Rosie's story. But she felt happy that Rosie seemed to be starting to become more open about talking to her, so she let it go. Sometimes Rosie wished that she could just open up and tell Melanie the truth. The knowledge that she was constantly lying made her feel far worse than the accrual thing that she was having to lie about. Maybe if it hadn't been David's child that she was carrying, she might have found it easier to be honest about being pregnant. Maybe her anxiety was an alarm system of some sort, now though. She realised now that she and David had pushed beyond the barriers by having a forbidden sexual relationship and that Melanie was actually an exceptional woman, who had tried her best to be as understanding about what was an intolerably painful situation for everyone concerned. Rosie's heart sank as she arrived on the ward with her overnight bag. The nurse showed her to her bed, and told her to wait to see the doctor. She tried reading some magazines that had been left by the previous patient, but all she wanted to do now, was to have this whole sorry business over and done with, and be freed from a responsibility that she just wasn't ready for. As soon as she had come out of the operating theatre, the responsibility would be taken away from her young shoulders, and she could start getting on with the rest of her life.

Having to decide whether to have an abortion or not when you are only fourteen is bad enough. Even women who are adults find it a difficult decision to make – add to that the question of whether the mother has serious mental illness or not, and one of the baby's parents is a family member, one has a potentially fraught situation at best, at the very worst it could turn into a life threatening situation for more than one person.................

After she had had the chance to recover from her ordeal, Rosie had never felt so relieved in her entire life. Now she could put all her worries to one side, and best of all, she had managed to get away with it – without Melanie finding out anything about it at all. Rosie always hated being in hospital, because of the lack of privacy. Thankfully, this time, she was in an all-female ward. But it was a gynaecology ward, where the women were all in there for a variety of different reasons.

Rosie found that the women were unfriendly towards her when she had come back from having her operation and the patient in the bed next to her was deliberately bullying her. In fact, she made Rosie feel distinctly uncomfortable, even though Rosie had tried to be friendly and talkative to her – considering how unwell Rosie was feeling after the operation, this was no mean feat.

"What are you in here for?" Rosie asked.

"I have just had another miscarriage." The girl told her. "It's my third one this year." Rosie suddenly understood.

"I'm so terribly sorry, …" she faltered.

"No you're not, sorry. You don't KNOW me. Anyway, why should you be sorry, when the reason that you are in here is because you've decided to kill your own baby, AND it's YOUR choice. Some of us would give everything to be able to make that choice." Rosie couldn't believe what she was hearing.

"If you must know, I didn't really have any choice in my situation, either. How old would you say I am?"

"What's that got to do with anything?"

"More than you'll know," said Rosie. "Seriously, how old would you say I was?"

"I'd say that you were sixteen."

"No, actually I'm fourteen" It was the girl's turn to look surprised.

"My appearance always gets me into trouble" Rosie told her. "Men always think that I am older than I am."

"Doesn't your mother advise you about appropriate dress?" asked the girl.

"No. She never has. I would just like to ask you a question. Which is worse, keeping a baby that you know you are not ready for, or not going through with it because you want the best thing for everyone concerned? What happens if it could affect the whole of your family? It's all too easy for people to be critical when they don't have the full knowledge of all the facts about the other person's situation. Secondly; it's none of their business, whatsoever. Thirdly, a person who is mentally ill is just as intelligent and capable of making a decision as the next person."

"Do you think you made the right choice?" she asked Rosie.

"I thought things through really carefully, and there was no other way I could have done this. I only wish there were" Rosie said, shaking her head. "You see, if I had gone ahead with the pregnancy full-term and had to give my baby away to someone else at the end of the nine months, I would have had to carry the guilt from that around with me for the rest of my life, and it's not just my life that would have been ruined by all of this, either."

"How can you make that choice about someone else's life?" asked the girl. "If you had had a scan, and something showed up on there, say the baby had Downe's Syndrome, or some other birth defect, or was seriously physically handicapped would you have decided to have an abortion on those grounds? Did you really think about all those couples who are desperate to have a baby of their own, and are in a much better position than you to look after it properly, just think, a nice house, a husband and wife together with everything except the one thing they are just longing for and just can't have? And then a little snippet of a thing like you comes along and decides to play God? If you ask me, there should be a new law made so that people who are mentally sick like you can be automatically sterilised, so that they don't pass on their peculiar behaviour to the next generation," she said angrily.

"I would have been glad to adopt your baby, if you had given me the chance. But there are too many selfish people in the world; I don't suppose you would even think about that."

"You see if I had gone ahead with the pregnancy full-term, and had to give your baby away to someone else after the nine months, I would have had to carry the guilt from that burden around with me for the rest of my life and it's not just my life that would have been ruined by all this, either. If your baby's father was a member of your own family, would you know what to do next, for the best?" Rosie asked.

"I know one thing is certain, that I wouldn't have an abortion whatever the circumstances. Who has the right to choose whether someone lives or dies? It's unnatural. It's completely against all the rules of nature. Let nature take its course. Life is a wonderful thing, and human life is completely sacred. No human being has the right to decide whether something else should live or die."

"Surely an individual has the right to make whatever decisions they see fit? As you so rightly say – it isn't anyone else's choice except theirs. What if you were so ill that you can't even look after yourself and so that means that it would be questionable whether you were a fit person to look after a child? Social services would definitely have to be contacted without a doubt. Anyway, I still don't see why all of this has got anything to do with you, at all."

"What about side effects from medication? I have already had a couple of miscarriages because of the medication that I am taking on a long-term basis then my psychosis becomes more difficult to handle. I wouldn't even consider risking the possibility of taking any medication at all while I was pregnant, not after what's happened to me the last time around. How would you know whether or not the medication wouldn't cause serious birth defects in your new baby?"

"I still think the most sensible thing would be to sterilise all female psychiatric patients, then they wouldn't become such a burden on society. I think that it should be much harder for people to get handouts from the state."

"Actually, I think that stinks." said Rosie. "Filling out all those complicated forms makes it almost impossible to be able to manage on your own without having a CPN to help you cope with all the paperwork. The moral of the story is then, that if you are not capable of filling in a few straightforward application forms for the DSS, then you definitely are not capable of being a fit parent. Whatever you think, I KNOW I made the right choice for everyone concerned in my situation." said Rosie angrily. "I am not prepared to discuss this any more. I'm supposed to be resting. I'm sorry you've had such a bad time, but it's hardly my fault, and not really my business, I don't want to talk any more." Rosie turned over on her side and pretended she was asleep, just to be able to put an end to this conversation.

Melanie had been well aware that somebody hadn't been telling her the whole truth. She couldn't remember the last time Rosie had even mentioned having any friends to hang out with, never mind staying away from home for overnight sleepovers. There was absolutely no doubt at all in Melanie's mind that everything was not as it should be, and nothing was as it seemed. Melanie wasn't game for having the wool pulled over her eyes any longer now either. Rosie had another thing coming. Two could play her game. Rosie must have thought that Melanie was completely naïve. Well this time, it was going to be Melanie who got the upper hand. As Melanie poured out her second cup of coffee, she could hear Rosie's key turn in the lock. "Ah…"Thought Melanie to herself. "Here we go…"

Melanie wasn't too sure how to respond to Rosie for the best. However, because Rosie looked so pale when she did turn up, Melanie began to be really worried.
 "How was the party, then?" she asked.
"Great, Mum"
"Did you stay up all night, haven't you had any sleep at all, young lady?" Melanie asked.
"No, actually, I haven't. Do you mind very much if we wait to talk until after I have had a chance to catch up on my sleep, first, at least?" replied Rosie.
"Not so fast young lady. You haven't been drinking alcohol on top of your medication, have you? You know perfectly well that you are not supposed to be drinking anything at all."
"I just had the odd drink, mum, nothing much. But I don't feel very well. Gosh, actually I'm feeling very sick" Rosie's colour changed dramatically, and she started to look decidedly green.

She rushed to the toilet. Melanie could hear her being very sick.
 But then Rosie started calling out to her.
"Rosie, what's the matter?"
"I can't stop bleeding"
"Is it your period?"
"No, this is much worse. There's blood pouring everywhere. HELP ME, please HELP ME."
"Shall I get the doctor?"
"No just the ambulance, quick, Oh God…"
"Can you open the door, Rosie?"

Melanie was concerned that if Rosie weren't able to open the door, then help wouldn't be able to get there fast enough. Rosie managed to open the door to let her mother in, but she was lying in a big pool of red blood looking as pale as death.

"What happened at the party?" Melanie asked as she helped her onto the sofa where she could lie down.

"Mum, I wasn't at any party last night." Melanie had thought as much. "I've been in hospital, I had an abortion yesterday."

"I beg your pardon?"

"I had to go through with a termination, you do understand, don't you?"

"Yes, I can, but what I don't understand, and what makes absolutely no sense to me whatsoever is that you didn't see fit to even mention to me that you were pregnant at all. I thought that we were supposed to be trying to give each other a fresh start – being able to trust each other. What happened to all that? I don't know if there's any hope left for us," said Melanie. "Here's the ambulance now. Do you want me to come with you this time, seeing that you obviously didn't want me to know anything about it at all? I have to tell you that I am extremely disappointed in you, and am not sure if we even have any kind of relationship at all, any more, not now, or ever."

PART 3
SONATA
Allegro

Melanie had definitely been pushed to the absolute limits, and had begun to reach the point of no return. What was even worse was that she felt so completely let down by everyone else in her family. This was total betrayal.

"There's nothing more that I can do any more now," thought Melanie. "I have tried and tried and tried and tried...but Rosie has gradually turned everyone completely against her, even me. She seems to be almost on some kind of vendetta. I can't do anything else anymore, not now this has happened. She's on her own" She didn't realise that she was doing Rosie a favour, by finally setting her free and allowing her to make her own way in life, as well as make her own mistakes.

"I'm looking after myself from now on" thought Melanie. "There's absolutely nothing more that I am able to do for her any longer. I'm not having her back in the house anymore when she comes out of hospital this time, that's it."

Rosie hadn't appreciated all the help and support that she had had from Melanie over the years. She just took it for granted that there would be somebody to look out for her, but not any more. She hadn't realised before how dangerous it was to take help from other people for granted. Would it be too late for her to make amends? What would she do without anywhere to stay after she came out of hospital? Rosie didn't want the social services to become too involved in her case because she thought that they would find out about her relationship with David. They were bound to. It was only a matter of time, but Rosie could no longer think up any more lies to back up her story.

She was determined that her only answer would be to go and search for her step-father, but she realised that she faced the moral dilemma of whether she told him that she had had an abortion, because it was his fault that she had got herself into this mess in the first place. Rosie decided that it was time to find out where her father was. He had become a taboo subject since she and Melanie had returned home, she was not allowed to talk about him. She could sense the tension between her and her mother every time it looked as if the conversation was going to take off in the direction of David's whereabouts, which still seemed to be a total mystery.

Rosie was mystified. How could David possibly reject her now? Why had he suddenly disappeared without trace? Well, she knew that it must be something to do with Melanie. Melanie had planned all this, right down to the very last detail. She felt that she'd been schemed against. She should have realised that actually, Melanie was trying to protect her from being hurt any further, but it was probably high time Melanie let go of Rosie completely and allowed her the freedom of her own independence. Even if Melanie was fearful of the mistakes Rosie would make in life without her guidance and wisdom, then she feared for her future. But sometimes the kindest thing to do under these circumstances is to allow people to make their own mistakes Although she was relieved to be out of hospital in many ways there were other aspects of being discharged that made her feel completely petrified. How could she be sure to make a full recovery when she didn't have anywhere that she could go to, to be able to focus on getting better? She was frightened as she faced the prospect of being homeless. She had no idea where to start looking for somewhere to live and equally that she didn't have the strength to go wandering the streets all by herself, which was what she was facing. Perhaps it could only be a good thing if she was able to reconnect with David. He would probably let her stay with him, even if only on a very temporary basis at least.

The problem was that Rosie couldn't remember what had happened between her and David in Amsterdam, because the E.C.T hadn't been the only thing affecting her memory.

The drugs had also started to block out other areas of her more recent past.

How much worse could things possibly get than a fourteen year old girl wandering the streets with nowhere to go, after having been discharged from hospital after an abortion? Rosie didn't know what she was more scared of, having to survive this trauma completely alone, or the prospect of spending her convalescence having to wander the streets without anywhere to call her own home.

Rosie had found it was not just difficult, but impossible to feel ok about being discharged from hospital. She knew she was on her own, this time. What was more, she'd been unable to get the right kind of follow-up support from Social Services, and she'd been in the situation of having to be uncooperative because she was scared of the implications of Social Services discovering her relationship.

Generally speaking, patients are misguided about the role of social services when it comes to helping them, especially in a situation where a child is involved. As soon as the word 'Social Services' is mentioned it seems to send some folk into a tizzy. They seem to fear the worst that once social services are brought onto the scene this means that they are under judgment that their baby will be taken away from them if they are seen to be an unfit parent. Of course no - one in their situation can ever live up to the high standards that they set for themselves. People so often forget, particularly if they are first time parents, that there is no such thing as the perfect parent, that it is ok to be just a "good enough" parent, and that most days, that's all any of us can hope for.

Rosie probably had a great deal more to fear than the majority of other people. She always felt that she was in the situation of having to make sure that she protected David from the possibility of discovery. The burden of having to keep the relationship from discovery was far too great for any fourteen years old to be expected to be able to handle.

If she hadn't been hearing voices, one could possibly have said that she was probably a remarkably strong   character, in fact, most folk with mental health problems have to be made of strong stuff, stronger stuff than ordinary people in the outside world. The outside world never gives you credit for that. It takes enormous willpower to be able to survive from one twenty-four hours to the next. It's no mean feat when someone is battling with a constant stream of negative thinking which gradually accumulates into "100 different ways to kill yourself" once every hour, every single day.

Maybe the role of the mentally ill in society at large has somehow become carnivalesque. Their role is upside-down, being viewed by the outside world as weaker, when in fact they are the ones who are the stronger as well as being extra special. It is so easy to view any kind of illness as a disadvantage. If the general approach towards illness could only be more positive, then the situation would end up being totally different.

As Rosie began her day wandering about the streets, with nothing but her thoughts for company, she realised that this was the first time in her entire life that she hadn't got a clue where she would be sleeping that night. The only helpful advice the hospital had been able to give her was that she would find information about homelessness at the Citizen's advice bureau, which was where she decided to head off to. They had actually been fairly helpful, and told Rosie that her best bet would be to head for the Salvation Army Hostel, or the local night shelter that could provide her with somewhere temporary to stay while she searched for a more permanent solution.

There were a number of issues that were bothering Rosie about becoming homeless, but her main concern was how she would be able to survive without much money coming in. Even people over the age of sixteen would have found it difficult enough to fill in the DSS forms without having any permanent address. So what in hell's chance did a fourteen years old kid stand?

It was, admittedly an extremely unusual situation for any fourteen year old to find themselves in, as the majority would have been able to continue to live at home. As far as Rosie could see, the only answer would be to locate David as soon as possible – but she had very little information to go on, it was rather like searching for a needle in a haystack. The only problem was that the residents at the Salvation Army Hostel were expected to vacate their rooms by 9 am in the morning, straight after breakfast and although they were given a full English fry-up and a steaming mug of tea to cheer them on their way, Rosie was concerned that she needed to find David as soon as possible, because she could see what little money she had would be spent on her tube fares. She hoped that David would at least be able to gibe her some money until she managed to sort something else out.

The only problem with walking around for hours is that somehow a person seems to spend a lot of time reflecting. This can be helpful, in most cases, but Rosie was trying to come to terms with the pain of grieving over her lost pregnancy, what had happened to her family, as well as being homeless on top of all of it. Somehow all the pain got muddled up inside her thoughts, added to which she was especially affected by her physical pain due to the after effects of her operation, not to mention the emotional pain of the bereavement she was suffering at the same time.

If she had been able to be more open about her relationship with her baby's father, she would probably have found that the Social Services would have been able to offer plenty of help and support, and she would have had someone to turn to. Since she had had the E.C.T treatment, she was disorientated in a way that she had never been before. Somehow, even though the psychosis was a terrible affliction to have to go through so regularly, the voices were almost a comfort to her. This time, though, she had felt a sense of becoming completely lost. As she was wandering the streets aimlessly, with no support from one single person in her family, no home, no secure place to lay her head, she was not only battling with the sense of loss that sprung from losing her unborn baby, but there were so many other issues to deal with that Rosie didn't even know where to start. Wandering around and around in circles, only not only made it all much worse, but the emotional pain became just as acute as the physical pain from the after-effects of her abortion. Sometimes Rosie wished that there were some kind of escape route from the prison that her own mind had created within herself. She felt even more unhinged since she had been on the psychiatric ward, because not only had she lost part of her identity, but the experience of being raped and losing the person who had hurt her, even though she hadn't been emotionally involved with him in the usual sense, had meant that she'd needed to block out more pain than ever. It was too much for even the most stable, mature adult to be able to cope with, let alone a schizophrenic fourteen-year old girl, who was still on the threshold of adolescence.

Rosie felt that she was at least fifty years old because of what she had to deal with. She knew she had had to grow up much faster than the average fourteen year old kid. As she walked through the park, she found that the images of the Magnolia tree had started to come back again, but the memories were so fragmented that she didn't even realise that the Magnolia tree was almost like the key to the door of her childhood past. It had been so many weeks since the treatment now that Rosie had just about given up hope of her memory returning. She almost wished that it had been her emotions that had been blocked out, not her memory, because, right now, she couldn't handle how she felt any longer. She wished she never had to feel. She didn't ever want to love anyone ever again, not ever – she didn't want to feel – maybe it might have been ok to feel love, but now she couldn't connect to her child self any longer, she just felt like her insides were almost like a huge block of ice that couldn't be moved. Something or someone had to either start hacking away at the block of ice, to break through, or pour so much warmth on to it that it would start to melt. But Rosie was so paralysed by the fear of being hurt that she was reluctant to even begin to think about connecting to other people. She had to protect herself, and now the biggest lesson that she had learnt so far, from damaging her family, was that she had to keep part of herself back, keep it back, just for her – not sharing all of herself with all and sundry any longer. But the next battle to be fought in her mind before the mindset could come crashing down was her sense of self, she had a major identity crisis on her hands, somehow there had to be a way to regain her lost childhood. Maybe once that happened, she could begin to hack her way through the block of ice, which would hopefully lose its power once it had been broken into splinters and fragments. If only she could find David, then maybe he would be able to help answer all these frightening questions. She had hoped to find her way over to the University at some point that day, but as the late afternoon turned into evening, she realised that her head was in too much of a muddle to continue the search for any longer that day. The other problem was that if you wanted to get a bed for the night at the night shelter, then you would have to make sure that you were there relatively early on, because the demand for a spare bed for the nigh was apparently extremely high, Rosie had already been alerted to this. So she thought it was probably better to find somewhere to stay and head for the university in the morning, maybe she might even have a clearer head once she had had the chance to sleep on everything.

Now her top priority had to be to find her way to the night shelter before it started getting too dark, as it was now early autumn, the nights were starting to draw in. Rosie was perturbed to discover that she was the only woman who was staying in the night shelter that evening. She didn't know which place was worse, the psychiatric ward, or the night shelter. There seemed to be very little to choose between them. But the hospital ward even seemed to be tantalisingly inviting in comparison to what was on offer at the night shelter now though. Rosie dreaded having to sleep here. It was a real eye-opener; she had never given homeless people much thought up until now. But she was in total shock as she realised the appalling degradation that homeless people faced, simply by the unhygienic conditions that they were forced to live in, just by not being able to have regular access to normal facilities such as a bathroom, that most of us fortunately have, but we take so many of our privileges for granted. Those of us who live in the Western world, don't often realise how privileged and lucky we are.

The hostel didn't provide meals, people were expected to be able to fend for themselves, but they did run a soup kitchen from there every evening, which meant that the residents could at least have a bowl of soup and some bread before settling down for the night. There were no single rooms, it was a case of everyone mucking in together, either sleeping en masse, in a big dormitory type room, or sharing with at least three others. As Rosie waited her turn in the queue for her soup, she had never felt so uncomfortable in her life. It was obvious that many of these people had been homeless for a considerable amount of time. There were quite a number of men there who looked as if they were beggars or tramps. Many of them were dressed in rags, and stank to high heaven. Obviously not many of them had even been able to have so much as a proper wash or even a bath for months. Rosie didn't want to communicate with anyone; she just wanted to get through this as fast as she could.

She felt sick as one of the men standing in the queue next to her started up a conversation. "How long are you here, luv?"

"It's not your business."

"I've been here six months now, thought I could find somewhere to live straight away, but, I thought wrong. We got chucked out of the squat."

"Were you squatters?"

"Yeah, sure we were. It was cosy, having a roof of sorts over our heads each night, somewhere to shoot the speed up our arms. But then the cops found out about shooting needles up our arms when they discovered needles in the school playground nearby, and guess who got blamed, and told to get the fuck out of here?"

"Were you using heroin?"

"We were doing speed. Would you like to try some spliff later?" he offered.

"No, thanks. So what's it like here?"

"It's cool, but you have to watch out that you don't catch nits. Some of these buggers, they are such filthy monsters. The nits love it here; they jump from one person's head to the next."

Rosie could feel her heart sinking lower and lower into a deep pit of despair.

How could she have been so selfish as to destroy her family? She hadn't realised how much Melanie had tried to help her survive, and the hard work she had done make a comfortable home. How Rosie longed to be back home with Melanie now.

If only she could make amends, but she feared it was just nothing but an impossible dream as she was facing this nightmarish situation, which was the starkest reality that Rosie had ever had to face in her young life. The porter came into the room to make an announcement: "If anyone wants to help do the soup run tonight, the van is leaving in fifteen minutes." Rosie jumped at the chance. As she helped the others load the van with paper cups, flasks of soup and blankets, she felt that she was making a valuable contribution to society, perhaps she could make a difference, do something useful.

The people she worked with that evening seemed to know every single corner in the city where there was someone sleeping rough. They knew everything about the people on the corners. Some of them had been sleeping rough for a few years, and had no intention of living their lives any other way. But although the hardship must be really difficult to bear in the middle of the winter, when you have been huddled under a thin blanket in the freezing cold conditions night after night, Rosie began to understand the reasons for someone wanting the freedom, as she watched so many different faces light up as they waited for the helpers to pass out cups of soup and a new blanket. She thought their faces almost glowed with happiness as the hot soup started to warm their freezing bodies. Maybe the rest of society had got all their values in life completely upside down. Perhaps it was time to reconsider what the important things in life really were. Rosie knew that she could begin to do this if she was able to find David, maybe she would have the chance to try to rebuild her connection with her family once more, if only that could happen, if only Melanie would be able to forgive and forget, she would be able to have a fresh start, and maybe the whole family could be happy again, one day. Not right now, though unfortunately, that only seemed to be a pipe dream.

Andante

The following morning Rosie decided to make as early a start as possible. She couldn't get away from the night shelter fast enough. Even though it was an experience that she would have preferred not to have to go through at all, she felt that she had learned some valuable lessons through it. Now all she could think about was to fulfil her quest, to find David as soon as possible.

She found the underground quite daunting, especially as she went down to the platforms on the long escalators. She knew she had to get to Camberwell. After about half an hour's walk from the tube station, she came to the university's art department. However, now she was actually facing the day of reckoning, she didn't think that she had the courage to actually go through with it; still she couldn't very well back out at this stage, not after having gone through all that trouble.

As she went into the main entrance of the art department, she could see there were lists of staff posted up on the notice boards. Rosie felt so relieved as she discovered the location of David's art studio. She decided to lose no time in going over there to find him. This had to be gone through; everything would be easier to deal with after this. Taking deep breaths, she knocked on the door of David's studio. There was no answer, but Rosie wasn't at all surprised, because it was still early in the morning. She tried the door handle. Surprisingly the door was unlocked. As she opened it, gingerly, she poked her head round it. The room was filled with easels and canvases. She walked round the room, shocked by the sketches. They were all of young women, which was nothing to be ashamed of initially, but Rosie was horrified by the fact that they were all nude. Every single one of them. That was when she got the biggest fright of her life, and found the painting.

Rosie went pale as she looked into Claire's eyes. The girl in the picture had the most beautiful long honey blonde hair. Her face was so full of expression; Rosie almost felt that the person in the painting was actually alive. She just stood, silently, looking at the painting, so transfixed that she hadn't noticed that there was someone else in the room.

"What are you doing?" A woman's voice said, making Rosie jump out of her skin. She realised that she was facing the woman in the picture.

"I'm sorry" Rosie hesitated. "I was only looking at the paintings. This one – it's you, isn't it?"

"Yes, but please answer my question, what are you doing here?"

"I'm looking for my step-father." Rosie told her.

"Well, I can't help with that; there isn't anyone here who fits that description, I am afraid."

"Would you help me find him, please, I know he teaches art here, his name is David." Claire hoped that she didn't look as startled as she felt.

"He should be here soon. He's coming to finish the painting this morning, I have another sitting. You are welcome to wait with me for him if you like. I had no idea that he even had a family." Mumbled Claire.

"Didn't you?" Rosie felt devastated at the prospect that David had been denying her very existence to make himself feel better, obviously. "He came to live at the university, after he broke up with my mother." She told Claire.

"Are your parents divorced, then?" asked Claire.

"No, just separated. I'm afraid it's entirely my fault."

"How can it be your fault?" asked Claire.

"Well, my mother has spent so many years looking after me when I have been ill. I have schizophrenia, and have spent loads of time in and out of mental hospitals. It's made life really difficult for the family."

"I still don't see how your mum and dad not getting on together is really your fault."

"Oh yes, it is, more than you realise." Rosie told her.

"Do you want to tell me about it?"

"No." Rosie became aware that she needed to keep something back, that she not only had to do everything to protect herself, but David as well. There was too much to lose once the real truth came out. Anyway, she didn't really know anything about the relationship between her stepfather and this woman, who could be anyone.

"Dad's painting you, isn't he?" Rosie said.

"Yes, it's a present for my mother's birthday. I think it's fantastic that your dad is such a brilliant artist. The other students love posing for him. His life drawing workshops are wonderful. Do you paint?"

"I'm not very good at anything, actually." Rosie told her.

"Oh come on, everyone is good at something." Said Claire. "What do you like at school?"

"I don't like school." Rosie said. "I hate it."

"Why?"

"Because I am always on my own. I don't have any friends." Claire felt like she was talking to a reflection of herself in a mirror.

"I went through that," she told Rosie. "You have never talked to anyone about this before, have you? Have you never talked to your mum about it?"

"There was never the chance to. Mum and Dad could never talk about anything without shouting and yelling at each other. Then my mum started to become more and more depressed. I did have one friend at school once, though. She was called Lorna."

"What happened to you and Lorna?" asked Claire.

"Do I have to talk about it, I don't want to talk about it, please don't make me…"

"Of course you don't have to talk about it if you don't want to, I just thought it might help." Rosie suddenly found that she felt that she had finally found a kindred spirit who would listen to her and not cast judgment on her.

"Well, Lorna was depressed. She had been for a long time. She was so angry. I never really found out why she was angry, she wouldn't tell me. I wanted to talk to her, to try to help; I wish I could have helped her before it was too late. But she wouldn't let anyone get close enough to her to be able to help her at all. Anyway, she must have tried every single trick in the book to kill herself, but nothing worked. One day she was mowing the lawn for her father, and decided that she couldn't cope with life a single moment longer; she grabbed the can of petrol and set fire to herself. It was nothing short of a miracle, but they got to her in time to save her life. However her face was so badly burnt that you couldn't recognise her for the disfigurement. She already had no confidence left. She kept wishing that she could be pretty again; 'how I was before my accident' she used to say. She could never face up to the truth; the truth of the matter was that it was no accident, that she had done it deliberately. Anyway, she went missing, after getting really upset with her parents for not being able to do anything more to help her. A few days later a passer by walked past the body of a young woman swinging from the branches of a tree, round and round, the body was suspended from the branches by a rope. My voices were a great comfort to me after that had happened."

"No wonder you must have felt like you were finally cracking up."

"I couldn't go to either of my parents, because they weren't communicating, the only way they could relate to each other was either by shouting the place down, or total silence. I feel so guilty about Lorna. I did try my best to help her get out and join in with everyone else. But the others were bullying me too, and I always felt on the outside of the group all the while. I know I don't have any confidence in myself, or any social skills."

"You know something…" Claire said, "You remind me so much of me. I was just like that at school. I hated sport, and no one could ever understand my passion for playing the piano. I always felt a freak about my appearance." Rosie looked shocked.

"But you're so beautiful,"

"It doesn't make you happy, you know, not necessarily, when you are good looking, you are always left wondering why people actually like you. My problem was that I always felt unlovable unless I could prove to everyone that I was special. I could do that with my music, but I always felt inferior about myself in every other way. My sister and I don't communicate anymore. She felt rejected like me, but it was worse for her, I think. She always felt that I was the one who got all the praise and attention because of being especially talented. I think she just felt too ordinary. She won't have anything to do with me now; I haven't seen her in years."

"When I had the E.C.T treatment to try to block out my voices, it made me feel terrible," said Rosie. "I didn't want to lose the voices, in fact, I would have preferred it if they had allowed me to keep them, and not interfered. The voices were the only things that I had to stop me from becoming too isolated. They kept me from going completely insane. But of course, no-one normal could possibly comprehend that. The treatment really stressed me out; I couldn't remember whole chunks of my past. But it seems that it's slowly starting to come back. I was scared of losing my childhood, my childhood is so important to me, it's one of the only times in my life that I was happy – when Mum and Dad were happy. What totally freaked me out was that I was scared that if my inner self had been killed off, then somehow my ability to give and receive love had been killed off too. I didn't feel human any more. I almost felt the same way after Lorna died. I didn't want to feel anything any more, the pain hurt too much."

"I was isolated, too. If you have to be exceptional at anything it involves cutting yourself off from everyone else to work, and I never had many friends either." Claire told her. "So you see, if you do take a chance and open up to someone eventually you'll find someone who'll understand better than you ever thought possible."

Rosie had been so confused by the pain of Jamie McBride's death, that the only way she could deal with the pain was to shut down her subconscious,   "Listen...'" continued Claire, "Do you know what I think? I think that you don't love yourself. If you don't love yourself, then how can you possibly love anyone else? I think you are very angry with yourself, but you need to stop that, and begin to be able to be less hard on yourself. But it takes a whole lifetime to learn how to love yourself. One's adolescence is only part of that journey. That's quite enough for any teenager to deal with; it takes wisdom and maturity, which only comes with experience. But you'll get there in the end – you'll see, believe me." Claire told her. "I've changed since I met David. He introduced me to some of his drug-taking friends. I hated it to start with, but one of them persuaded me that drugs could actually help make you feel better, and persuaded me to try them, now I've realised that may be I've been too prejudiced about so many things, that maybe I need to keep more of an open mind, instead of writing things off."

Rosie wasn't quite sure how, but what Claire had been describing to her had somehow meant that she was conscious, that some of her lost memory was finally beginning to wake up. The pain of dealing with Jamie's death had meant that it was easier to bury it into the subconscious, rather than have to face it immediately and deal with it there and then. Only now, when she had had the first opportunity to open up to someone else, was she able to voice what she had been carrying around inside her all this time. Both women were so engrossed in their conversation that they hadn't noticed that David was standing in the doorway of the art studio.

Allegro Vivace

The studio was filled with a deathly silence, apart from the sound of one of the windows, which had been blown open by the wind. Banging to and fro, as the heavy rain pelted against it, sounding like Rosie's pounding heartbeats as she faced David for the first time since she had had the abortion. David was sopping wet, with raindrops dripping from his wet hair and clothes.

"Darling…" he started, as he approached Claire, but Rosie had assumed that he was talking to her. David's eyes fell on Rosie. "Who are you, and what do you want?" Rosie couldn't believe this.
"Dad, it's me – Rosie."
"I don't know who you are." David glowered at her, then he walked over to Claire, putting a protective arm lovingly around her, but Claire pushed him away, shocked by his response to Rosie. "I'm sorry I 'm a bit late, my darling." David told her. "I hope you haven't had to wait too long, my love." Rosie cringed when she heard those words. It had never occurred to her that David might be involved with Claire in a relationship context. But she hadn't expected to have to deal with the prospect of having her entire existence being totally denied by her stepfather. Well, she'd put up with quite enough of the betrayal and the lies now. She certainly wasn't prepared to cope with anymore of David's lies. She'd lost too much already.

"Why are you still here? Would you mind just leaving?" David asked Rosie. "What's wrong, David?" Claire asked reassuringly.
"I don't know this person. I have absolutely no idea what she wants." David told Claire. Rosie jumped as she saw the sudden flash of lightening as it streaked across the grey sky. The rumble of thunder followed a split second afterwards; she noticed the sky growing blacker and blacker as it filled with the dark rain clouds. "I was pregnant." Screamed a voice that seemed to be almost a part of Rosie but was somehow still separate. "I had an abortion two

weeks ago, and I killed OUR baby, YOUR baby, YOURS AND MINE. I'm a MURDERER"

Rosie screamed out at the top of her lungs…

."Murderer… murderer…murderer…murderer…" her voices started echoing, resounding around in her head, growing louder, louder and louder in response to her overwrought emotions, echoing the guilty thoughts that had been swirling around inside her head ever since she had first made the decision to have the abortion. Rosie was shaking with the suppressed rage that she'd buried in her unconscious mind for months, ever since her best friend had committed suicide, somehow, now she knew that she had told everything about her secret past to yet somebody else who couldn't be trusted, having the chance to let everything out into the open meant that she now had the chance to free herself from her frozen anger that had piled up and up and up. But all Rosie was left with now was the gnawing pain that she had been too scared to face up to, ever since Lorna had died, and she had run into David's warm arms. As she watched the streaks of lightening across the grey skies outside, the previously unacknowledged pain gnawed at her, gripping her from the inside out, she'd managed to run from it so far, ever since Lorna's death. But now she was stripped bare of the warmth of David's love, and found she could run, but could no longer hide.

She couldn't cope with the mounting fury that was raging around as she was trying to handle years and years of emotional baggage. She couldn't look David or Claire in the eye. As her eyes wandered around the studio, they landed on the worktop surface where the art students made their own canvasses. That was when her eyes fell on the hammer. She wanted to destroy the pseudo beauty created by the artistic surroundings.

A thing of beauty is a joy forever. The stark contrasts between the positive energy of creativity, the artistic genius as it somehow became drawn into a fight against the destructiveness of the deep, dark depression with its inactivity, and unproductiveness as it destroyed everything in its path. The positivism of the creative energy coming from the dedication and commitment involved in creating works of artistic genius, somehow became swallowed whole in the war against pride at achieving something magical and beautiful, as the mind starts to accept the positive energy instead of struggling with the low sense of self worth, self denial, and self hate which swamps somebody struggling to survive everyday life with severe depression and psychosis.

But can the psychosis become a gateway for creativity and positive energy, the arts open up the opportunity to release the emotions using new insights and everyone has the chance to find their own personal fulfilment when it comes to self-expression. Once the dormant emotions have found a twisting pathway for their release, the pathway will lead the way, for the blind to find their sight, the deaf to hear, and the darkness of depression will be destroyed to be replaced by the radiant light of the true person who is just longing to be freed from their prison of self inflicted destructiveness.

Her voices told her to go over and pick up the hammer. CRACK went the next flash of lightning, as she brought her hammer down on the art table, smashing the jars filled with water all over the floor. Smithereens of broken glass everywhere as she swept through every object in sight in her wake. FLASH, went the lightening as she could feel the pain inside her, for the pain of the screaming sound of the cries of her unborn child, as she swung the hammer backwards and bought it forwards again, as she smashed one window after the other. David and Claire were too terrified to attempt to try to stop her, but as she dropped the hammer, and sank to the floor, sobbing and sobbing, David made a lunge for her, escorting her out of the studio and running with her and Claire to the car. Everything was starting to happen so quickly that no one realised that David was completely drugged and unfit to drive; it didn't become evident until he started driving down the street at top speed.

David could hardly concentrate on the road in front of him as Rosie screamed at the top of her lungs. "**Liar**...liar ...liar...You LIAR...HOW COULD YOU?" He was terrified as Rosie suddenly started punching him in the stomach, harder and harder and harder. Suddenly he took both hands off the steering wheel as he doubled up in agony, the car swivelled around in a circle. All anyone could remember was a feeling of spiralling down and down and down, downwards into the complete blackness of total oblivion.

EMPTINESS. BLACKNESS.

L'APRES MIDI D'UNE FAUNE
The Afternoon Of A Faune, Claude Debussy

Survival. This mental health game everyone is playing is all about survival. Survival, as one rolls the dice to play the next stage of the game of Monopoly. There is inevitability going to be some losers in the mental health game. It's a bit like a game of chess. But the mental health game can become like the analogy of winning and losing. It depends how the players manage to approach it. The winners can also be the ones who society considers to be the losers. Anyone who has the courage to survive from one twenty-four hours to the next, who dares to survive the struggle of trying to decide whether to give up the fight and end one's life, or press forwards, onwards and upwards has the right to celebrate the victory, for they are victorious. Not defeated.

How anyone could have survived the car crash at all is beyond belief. But there were two survivors. It was nothing short of a miracle that there was only one death. But she was still very much alive.

She hadn't really lost; she'd not given in to the years of fighting her own personal war with life. This was just like a game of Monopoly or Chess; she had to be a winner.

Rosie had her peace of mind now, at long last.

David was a winner. He had been forced to tell the truth about himself for the first time in his life. Claire had decided to take him to a narcotics anonymous meeting, when he finally told her that he never wanted to take drugs again in his entire life, after losing Rosie. And she believed every single word.

Claire's heart swelled with pride as she watched David stand in front of the sea of faces in the silent room, you could have heard a pin drop.

"My name is David," he faltered, glancing at Claire. "And I 'm an addict."

Was he really David standing there telling the truth? He couldn't even remember his own personality any more, not after pretending to be somebody else ever since he and Melanie had separated. Their whole marriage had been based on lies, lies, lies and yet more lies. Melanie had known absolutely nothing whatsoever about David's addiction.

She had been trapped in a web. Perhaps David had been blatantly lying to himself that he was self – medicating rather than face up to the uncomfortable truth that he, and he only was the one totally responsible for tearing his family to pieces. There were so many regrets.

But the biggest regret of all was his relationship with Rosie, and everything it had ended up costing him in the past .Losing Rosie was the biggest regret of all. It was too late to change that now, He felt powerless. But anyway, at least, he might have learnt something from his past behaviour, and put it to good use to change the future. His and Claire's future. Claire was the only thing that he had left that was worth living for.

His love for her made him want to be a better person. She was so pure, so beautiful, that she coaxed the truth out of him, because she was so special, she deserved that much from him, at the very least.

She was so lovely, that she made him feel that his insides had been littered up by the filth of his lies. , And the deepest shame that living a life totally based on being totally incapable of being able to be honest, especially with his own wife. His relationship with Melanie had to have had something basic missing from it. David figured that any romance had been killed off a long time ago, and it had been because of the situation of having a family member who was struggling with a severe mental illness.

He never really blamed Rosie. But he certainly began to see himself in a different light, and now that he was standing up in front of all those people because of this beautiful young girl who was the love of his life, he knew he owed it to her he didn't deserve her. Looking at her standing there, watching him, her eyes full of love, longing and hope, bought feelings of the deepest shame imaginable, feelings of shame cutting through the deep scars of his heart which he had shut down from long ago, because he used the drugs to cover the fact that there was too much pain inside for him to cope with.

His biggest fear now was that Claire would leave him. Especially, as soon as she knew the truth. The thought of being without her was much too painful to deal with. He thought that he would find it easier to give up taking drugs forever than go for a whole day without Claire.

He hadn't meant to lie to Claire when he stood up in front of all those people. He meant what he said from the bottom of his heart and the very depths of his soul. It was a privilege to be able to savour her beauty – it made him want to keep his promise to her Lost in the magic of that transformational moment, neither of them had any inkling that they were heading down a very slippery slope with no regard for the consequences.

Can a leopard change its spots? "Once an addict, always an addict" is this the truth? Even though many addicts have every intention of giving up their addiction once they realise the pain they are inflicting onto their nearest and dearest, they are fighting against all the odds – Sometimes they come out fighting, sometimes not.

The universal thing they all have in common is that when they say they want to stop taking drugs forever is that the majority of them really mean it.

But then things happen. It becomes easier for them to stay in the place that they have always been branded – liars. The word spirals out of control, propelling towards causing another tragedy. Tragedy has so many meanings, the lost chance of transformation, and the lost opportunity to prove oneself against all the odds ....Sometimes unconditional love is enough to help the other person achieve everything they hope and dream for.

Sometimes it just isn't enough.

Claire was deluding herself - she was entangled into the spiders web being weaved, hanging onto its threads, like a fly being ready to be swallowed whole by the spider waiting for the opportunity to leap onto its bait. Maybe Claire was an easy target. It seems that anyone who has problems with low self-esteem becomes party to playing the role of victim.

Claire had already become David's victim. She had been swept along by the powerful force of her emotional entanglement to the point of almost living under an illusion. She knew David would do anything for her – absolutely anything. The meeting heralded new beginnings. Perhaps both of them had found the hope for a better tomorrow, after they walked out of the meeting, All Claire knew was that she desperately longed to give David the chance of the lasting happiness which he had a perfect right to, and, which for now had been passing him by. As they walked home she hoped so much that she would be the one who helped David to realize his dreams.

But the illusion was about to be broken, and they were to plunge into an earth shattering reality that neither of them had envisaged. For, the truth was that they had already started spiralling and sliding down the very slippery slope the minute they walked into the house later that afternoon.

Being together was the only thing that mattered right now. All they both wanted was to seek refuge and comfort in the warmth of each others bodies, curled up against each other, comforting each other in the warmth.

The web was spinning faster and faster.............

The Sorcerer's Apprentice.

Four weeks later, David's situation hadn't changed at all since the meeting. During the meeting, he had felt inspired, standing up in front of the others, feeling that he was capable of anything.

But he found that changed the minute he returned into his normal environment. Almost as soon as he had walked through the front door, in fact. Old habits die hard. It had been one thing making promises up there. The reality of the situation was quite another. He had felt so transparently honest standing there. But now the illusion had been smashed, and he found himself back in the reality of the here and now.

It had only been a matter of one short week before he had broken his promise to Claire. After the first few days of being without drugs, he had begun to experience the shakes, and went into cold turkey. He was still being deceitful to Claire, who thought that he was clean. He was lying through his teeth. He was still putting drugs into Claire's drinks to persuade her to have sex with him, because he found that was the only way he could cope with the cold turkey.

Claire had noticed a change In David's behavioural patterns almost as soon as he had started to come off the drugs. At first she thought that he had the 'flu, as he was walking around the house with his nose streaming constantly, and becoming hot and cold, which made her think he was suffering some kind of sickness, and led her to believe that he had a viral infection..

As time went on, however, different symptoms began emerging, that made her realise it was something else. He kept having to disappear to the toilet for long periods of time, where she could hear the sound of him retching, as he vomited, until he finally emerged, looking completely drained of all energy.

But it was the effect on his mental stability, causing serious episodes of prolonged delusions, resulting in David becoming totally confused which gave Claire the most cause for concern.

One morning Claire came into the bedroom where she found David freaking out. Claire couldn't take any more. Claire suspected David might be suffering from paranoia, but she hadn't realised that what she was actually witnessing, i.e. the classic withdrawal effects of somebody who was in the recovery process of prolonged drug misuse.

She wanted to encourage David to stick through this tough time, even though she was suffering from worrying herself stupid about him.

He used that fact to his advantage, and managed to convince her that he was completely clean, when in actual fact, the delusions and freak-outs that he was experiencing were so unbearable that he had resorted to his old tactics of lies. All hope had flown out of the window

As David had flushed all the evidence down the toilet, when he had his head in the toilet bowl being sick, they had run out of their supply of drugs, and had no money to fall back on to buy more.

"What are we going to do?" Claire asked David. "I can't go on like this any longer. I HAVE to get hold of the dope. I can't bear to see you suffer like this any longer. What the hell's the point of going through all this pain and mental agony, when all it's ending up doing is making you sick? You MUST let me do something to help."

"But I'm doing this for YOU, for US. " David lied. "You have no idea what a total fool I will feel if I EVER touch that evil crap again I certainly don't want to play the hypocrite by encouraging you to take them as well as me."
"You aren't." Claire told him. "It's MY choice to do this, remember, no-one has ever been able to force me to do anything. I'm a grown woman, I make up my own mind; Anyway, you've done me a favour; Drugs are such fun. I can't think of a better way to help myself feel better about myself."

"What about your piano? " David said." The piano has only ever been a mask I hide behind. Sure it makes me feel good, for a while, but then I realise that I am dealing with my low self-esteem. When I take the heroin it makes me feel SO good about myself, that I know t I'm ok. I know it's the answer to stop feeling crap about myself."

"But don't you find that you spiral back down into depression again after a while?" David was concerned and curious. He realised that Claire had started becoming SO vulnerable. He knew that she had gone beyond the danger point with her addiction. He felt that if only he could point her back towards the direction of her musical talent, that that would provide the gateway to a way out of becoming addicted to the point of exceeding the danger mark.

Unfortunately, though, she already started careering down the slippery slope as if it were an avalanche. "I hope you realise that selling all our stuff is going to be the only way that we're going to be able to raise enough cash to survive, man."

"I thought you were off the dope?" Claire suddenly realised that she was being deceived. Being drawn into his pattern of thinking was part of the manipulation process. She knew that she was being manipulated, so that he would get away with being able to go back onto drugs if the withdrawal symptoms became too uncomfortable for him to deal with at all. Manipulation was his survival kit. Who was he fooling? He was certainly succeeding in fooling Claire, who felt sickened by the fact that he was preying on her pity. She knew she would end up loathing him if he carried on treating her like this. She had to get away.

The following morning, it was Claire's turn to spend half the morning with her head in the toilet. She had woken up feeling really sick. David responded to the situation in exactly the same way that Claire had done to his. He thought it was injecting that had caused her to feel so bad, but Claire suspected it was something else." I must get to the Doctor." She told David. "I feel so peculiar. I've never felt this bad before."

"You can't go anywhere in that state." David lied to her. "I'm going to go and see if I can get my hands on some more dope. That will make you feel better soon;" " Can I have the house key while you go out then?" Claire asked.

"No, sweetie, I'm afraid not." David told. "Well, if that's the case, then I will just have to come with you." Claire told him." No way, do you have any idea of the trouble you will get me in if you find out where I go to get the stuff?" "Don't you think I have the right to know?" Claire asked. "Listen, you are getting into a dangerous space. Man- "David told her. "You just don't have a clue how nasty these guys are, or could get if they think they have been dobbed in. "

"Is one of your suppliers that black guy I saw you pass a packet to down the pub?" Claire challenged him. "If I tell you anything, anything at all, it is going to be a BIG BIG risk to both of us." David told her." Things have got so much worse since the niggers started to do dope on the streets. It never used to be as bad as that when I was first dealing as a lad. The niggers have fucked everything up in this country. They are the ones who are responsible for all the crimes, but it's US who get dobbed in and have to answer to the police and the rest of society. The niggers are the ones who are responsible for all the shootings and gang shootings that have been going on round here, lately."

"Just listen to yourself." Claire said, angrily. "You are turning into such an offensive racist pig. You should hear yourself." Mr perfect"-, I don't think so. I've been as sick as a dog this morning, and need a doctor. I really don't think that you love me anywhere near as much as you say that you do, otherwise you would be thinking about looking after me. It's turning out to be the other way round these days." "Shut the fuck up." David was now starting to yell." No – I won't be spoken to like that ." David slapped her face, leaving Claire reeling backwards as she felt the impact of his slap and rushed out of the front door locking it behind him. It suddenly dawned on Claire that she had probably just become the latest victim of domestic violence. Well, there was no way she was going to turn into one of those women who kept leaving and then coming back time and time again for more, listening to the cheap promises of their partners who would say "I'll never do it again, babe." Claire knew only too well that once a man had hit you the once, there was no turning back.

That was the wake- up call, the signal to get out.

But for now, she was locked in the house and she had no idea how long she was going to be left alone for.

David didn't come back for three whole days.

The Girl With The Flaxen Hair

Claire spent the longest three days of her life plotting and planning the escape route from her prison. At least, that was the way it felt to be locked in somebody else's house against her will. She knew that she would have to make a run for it as soon as David opened the door. She felt sad, because she also realised David's motives behind his bizarre behaviour.

She was fully aware that he had locked her in because he was absolutely terrified of losing her - but the fear of loss was driving her towards loathing him even more than lying to her had done. She felt suffocated and smothered. She needed room to breathe, and he was suffocating her so much, especially with all the anxiety that he was piling onto her because of worrying about his health. She was beginning to feel as if she didn't have her own identity any more - that her true personality was slowly disintegrating.

It never occurred to her that it might have been the effects of the heroin addiction that were making her lose her identity. What didn't help anything was the oppression she had been subjected to by being forced to stay in the house with no means of getting out. She had no choice but to spend most of those three days sleeping, simply to pass the time, but she found herself awake, sitting bolt upright, waiting to hear the key turn in the lock, so that she could bolt as soon as David returned.

Eight O' clock the following morning it happened – finally.

Suddenly, David was standing in the hallway, and Claire found her arms being held above her, pinning her against the wall. How she managed to break free from his grasp, she never knew, but by some miracle, she managed to make it out of the front door. Stopping suddenly, as soon as she was outside, she was gasping for breath; as she had started to panic breathe.

David crept up behind her, pushing her to the ground. Claire was so pale, "You really think I am going to let you get away, don't you?" He shouted at her, then the punches started coming. Thump. Thump, thump, thump. He punched her stomach, making her double up with the sheer agony and tension inflicted onto her by the one person she thought loved her. Now she knew that it wasn't so.

Claire lay on the ground sobbing and sobbing, "Please just let me get to the doctor, I WILL come back. I never said I was leaving you."

"You bitch, there is no way YOU'RE going anywhere."
Suddenly Claire felt somebody pull her long blonde hair. David had grabbed hold of the beautiful, long, honey coloured hair that he had stroked so gently once, not so very long ago – and was dragging her back into the house by its roots. Claire's screams attracted the attention of a male passer-by .By a miracle, David let go of Claire when he saw the unwelcome sight of a stranger coming to interfere, and went back into the house, leaving Claire shaken.
"Are you all right?" asked the stranger.
"Please call the police." Claire sobbed." I think he's trying to kill me.

Half an hour later a policeman and policewoman were helping Claire up. But David was refusing to let them come inside the house.
"What do you want to do?" the policewoman asked Claire.

"I'm never going back to him." Claire told her." My things are still in there."

"Don't worry, my colleague will take you to the hospital, for the once over, and I'll get a few things for you now, then you can come back for the rest, later." said the male policeman.

"But he's got my piano in there." wailed Claire." He was talking about selling everything before he went crazy."

"We can't move the piano for you today." The policeman told her. "We'll get a few things sorted out like your clothes, but you will have to sort out the rest for yourself."

They escorted Claire to the police car; the policewoman drove her to her mother's house. Claire was forced into the position of living at her mother's place-this was originally only a temporary arrangement, until she got her head together enough to be able to look for a home of her own.

As it turned out, though – it was the best option available to her, as she was able to be protected and supported in a way that just couldn't 't have happened had she been left to fend for herself completely alone. The situation was difficult enough as it was.

When Claire woke up the next morning, in her own bed – in her old room, surrounded by all her favourite things that she had kept since she was a little girl, her collection of soft teddy bears – a huge bean bag on the floor, and her pine wooden rocking chair, she was lulled into a false sense of security- almost to the point of becoming delusional. Her illusion of almost perfect happiness was broken that very same morning.

Almost as soon as she was up and dressed, she had started feeling extremely sick. Her mother offered her love and comfort in the form of a mug of hot sweet tea, but the very thought of having to drink anything at all, sent Claire retching. She sat at the breakfast table with her mother, who sat reading the newspaper while she ate a light brown boiled egg and soldiers, made of white home-made bread spread with butter, which had always been Claire's favourite meal ever since she was a little girl. "Do you fancy an egg, dear" her mother asked. "I can try." Claire replied. So her mother set about preparing another egg. Unfortunately, this was also doomed to dismal failure, in spite of all the loving kindness that had accompanied its preparation.

"Is everything all right?" Claire's mum asked, hesitatingly, extremely anxious at the sight of Claire growing so pale she was beginning to look as white as a sheet. "No, Mum, I think I am going to be sick." she responded, rushing to the bathroom. That was when the phone calls started coming.

Claire could hear the piercing, sound of the phone ringing and ringing and ringing as she flushed the toilet bowl, and washed her face in the icy cold, clear water. She picked up the phone, unprepared to face what she was about to face." Hello?" It was then she realised David was crying on the other end of the line.

"Why have you left me?" He sobbed –"I can't live without you – my heart is breaking. If you don't come back I'll kill myself."

Claire's automatic response to hearing David's voice was to put the phone down without speaking a word to him. Shaking like a leaf she sat down. The phone calls kept coming over the next couple of months. Claire managed to avoid answering the phone as much as possible most of the time. One evening, however – she had no choice but to answer it. "Hello is that Claire?" a female's voice she didn't know was on the other end. "Yes – who am I speaking to?" "This is Anna." "Do I know an Anna?" Claire asked." Yes. I have someone here who wants to talk to you. Shall I pass you on to them?" said Anna. "All right – I'm not sure who you are though." replied Claire.

"I'll hand them over to you." Anna said. "What are you going to do about collecting all your things from the house?" said David.

Claire couldn't believe David would have stopped so slow to manipulate his own sister into making a phone call on his behalf, when it must have been obvious to anyone in their right mind that Claire wanted nothing more to do with them. But she had forgotten that David WASN'T in his right mind.

Claire put the phone down immediately. She'd already had the results from her pregnancy test, which had turned out positive – and had gone ahead and booked the termination. She was determined to go ahead. She'd spent all this time fighting to leave David – and having a baby made her feel totally trapped – unable to escape from this traumatic situation for the whole of the rest of her life. Since she had lost her piano Claire had started to lose all her confidence, to a much greater extent than ever before. She knew she HAD to play again, before she could start to feel any better, or feel anything at all, come to that. That was the only reason her life was worth living. First of all, though, she needed to get through this abortion in one piece, without cracking under the pressure, which was mounting steadily.

The day of the termination found Claire lying on the trolley, dozing off after her injection, confident that when she woke the nightmare would be over, and she could get on with the rest of her life.

"Today is the first day of the rest of your life". Claire remembered someone saying to her. She certainly felt that way now. She was surprised at how quickly they let her go home. Perhaps too quickly, as she started to get stomach cramps and began bleeding heavily once she was at home. Sure enough she was back in the hospital having to go through the whole process yet again. To add insult to injury she discovered that she had been carrying twins…

She felt like a serial killer on the loose…

Claire's mother hadn't told her that David had started turning up, looking for her. She knew Claire had quite enough on her plate as it was, but had made the best possible choice under the circumstances.

Mrs Powell longed for her daughter to find true happiness – goodness knows, she deserved it, after everything she had gone through. If they could get rid of David – then maybe, just maybe that might be possible. But however right one's circumstances are as human beings, one can only start to be happy if one truly desires to be so – then one can, and WILL.
You'd better believe it.

After Claire's departure, David had lost all sense of being any kind of a human being. He couldn't forgive himself for the way he had treated Claire at the end of the relationship. He hadn't meant to become violent – but he hadn't been able to get his hands on any drugs since he had been out of money, and it was driving him crazy. He always believed, in spite of everything that had happened over the last few terrible months that Claire would come back to where she belonged- with him in their house.

That was just David's perception of the situation – Claire knew there was no way she belonged there. David spent every single waking moment in denial believing that she was going to come back to him. That was the only reason why he hadn't sold any of her things up until then.

His travels had taken him to the Samaritans who had told David that they were worried that Claire was pregnant. Now his prime concern was that he would find her in time to stop her from killing his child. What gave women the right to think that they could play God when it came to giving life? They had absconded all their responsibilities when they had been irresponsible enough not to make sure they were protected enough in the first place. Surely such a decision shouldn't be made until both people had sat down and talked about it together – at least had the chance of having their opinion HEARD. For crying out loud, it was nothing short of criminal just to make a decision to take away a person's rights to make an informed choice, and just go ahead without even telling someone.

David hadn't bargained for how bad this made him feel, now the truth was dawning on him, that she hadn't thought enough of him to even tell him she was pregnant in the first place. He couldn't even bring himself to paint since she had gone. He was too churned up inside. He must be so evil, that no woman would ever want to carry his child, squirming around inside her for nine whole months. But David didn't have any idea that he needed to grieve , not just for losing Claire, but for the death of two children (he didn't have a clue that potentially three unborn children were now robbed of any chance of life, and all his hopes and dreams had been stolen from him without his knowledge or consent.

All he could think of was getting revenge for all the tormenting guilt, grief and unbearable pain that was gnawing away inside him as he was going through the scars of dealing with his bereavement. And he knew just how he was going to do that.

He had managed to find out that Claire had had an abortion, and now was going to be HIS moment – his moment had come to get full revenge, and back in control. He would sell all of Claire's things and make a special deal out of selling her piano- the bitch deserved everything she got for going ahead and murdering his child.

The day Claire came home after her second operation, she was still struggling to come to terms with things herself. She had never intended to answer the phone, but was now so drained and tired that she no longer cared who was on the other end in quite the same way any more. It took far too much effort to consistently ignore the phone.

"You Murderer." said the voice.
It was THE VOICE. The dark, scary voice continued.......
"I have robbed you now, in the same way that you have robbed me. You don't have your piano any more. I have

sold all your things, and sold your piano– so , now you know how it feels to have everything you ever dreamed of stolen from you."

Claire's first instinct was to find her needle and make herself feel better by injecting herself. She plunged the needle into her arm and promptly passed out, she never regained consciousness.

Epilogue

What must life be like without beauty? Without the beauty of magical sounds to listen to, to transport one away from the darkness in one's soul. Without being able to express one's emotions through sound, to break free from the monotony of everyday existence by experiencing the variety freely available through the joys of music?

To be able to lose oneself and break free from the every day stresses and strains by experimenting and playing with different tones shades, colours on a canvas, experiencing the removal of all anxiety as one moves the brush up and down a canvas covered in every single colour of the rainbow.

Experiencing the wonderful magic of art and sound through nature........ The unique sunsets at the end of every summer's day..... That magical rainbow...............

Life without artistic expression has no meaning. Being able to experiment with the arts of any discipline imaginable has to be the best cure and the way forward for the future for those learning about, and struggling to overcome a mental illness.

Better than slowly being poisoned by chemicals damaging one's body. Maybe some have no choice but to carry on taking medication, and certainly no decision should be made without consulting the doctors who are caring for you, but they should be helping you discover your self worth and potential as well, and what better way than prescribing the arts?

For it is by discovering and unlocking one's raw talents, that the cycle of self destruction is broken forever.

THE END

ARTS AND MENTAL HEALTH ORGANISATIONS.

Creative Routes
Camberwell Leisure Centre
5, Artichoke Place.
Camberwell
London SE5

0207 77330 24

Lost Artist's Club.
c/o City Arts
Unit 7
Newdigate Street.
Radford.
Nottingham
NG7 4 FD

City Arts
Provident Works
Newdigate Street .
Radford.
Nottingham
NG7 4FD

MENTAL HEALTH CHARITIES AND ORGANISATIONS

Central Notts MIND
Concorde House
12/14 St John's Street.
Mansfield.
Nottingham.
NG 18 1QK
06123 658040

RETHINK
25 a Outram Street
Sutton In Ashfield
Nottinghamshire
NG17 4BA
01623 466300

Speaking Up
Nottinghamshire Advocacy Alliance
DBH House
Carlton Square
Nottingham
NG4 3BP
0115 9408591

John Storer Clinic - Alcohol and Drug Addiction Rehab Unit
115 The Ropewalk
Nottingham
NG1 5OU
0115 941 46446979

Making Waves
39/41 Handel Street
St Ann's
Nottingham
Ng3 1J2